The Human Brain during the Third Trimester 225- to 235-mm Crown-Rump Lengths

This eleventh of 15 short atlases reimagines the classic 5-volume *Atlas of Human Central Nervous System Development*. This volume presents serial sections from specimens between 225 mm and 235 mm with detailed annotations. An introduction summarizes human CNS developmental highlights around 6.5 months of gestation. The Glossary (available separately) gives definitions for all the terms used in this volume and all the others in the *Atlas*.

Key Features

- Classic anatomical atlases
- Detailed labeling of structures in the developing brain offers updated terminology and the identification of unique developmental features, such as germinal matrices of specific neuronal populations and migratory streams of young neurons
- Appeals to neuroanatomists, developmental biologists, and clinical practitioners
- A valuable reference work on brain development that will be relevant for decades

ATLAS OF
HUMAN CENTRAL NERVOUS SYSTEM DEVELOPMENT
Series

Volume 1: The Human Brain during the First Trimester 3.5- to 4.5-mm Crown-Rump Lengths

Volume 2: The Human Brain during the First Trimester 6.3- to 10.5-mm Crown-Rump Lengths

Volume 3: The Human Brain during the First Trimester 15- to 18-mm Crown-Rump Lengths

Volume 4: The Human Brain during the First Trimester 21- to 23-mm Crown-Rump Lengths

Volume 5: The Human Brain during the First Trimester 31- to 33-mm Crown-Rump Lengths

Volume 6: The Human Brain during the First Trimester 40- to 42-mm Crown-Rump Lengths

Volume 7: The Human Brain during the First Trimester 57- to 60-mm Crown-Rump Lengths

Volume 8: The Human Brain during the Second Trimester 96- to 150-mm Crown-Rump Lengths

Volume 9: The Human Brain during the Second Trimester 160- to 170-mm Crown-Rump Lengths

Volume 10: The Human Brain during the Second Trimester 190- to 210-mm Crown-Rump Lengths

Volume 11: The Human Brain during the Third Trimester 225- to 235-mm Crown-Rump Lengths

Volume 12: The Human Brain during the Third Trimester 260- to 270-mm Crown-Rump Lengths

Volume 13: The Human Brain during the Third Trimester 310- to 350-mm Crown-Rump Lengths

Volume 14: The Spinal Cord during the First Trimester

Volume 15: The Spinal Cord during the Second and Third Trimesters and the Early Postnatal Period

The Human Brain during the Third Trimester 225- to 235-mm Crown-Rump Lengths

Atlas of Human Central Nervous System Development, Volume 11

Shirley A. Bayer

Joseph Altman

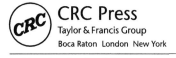

CRC Press
Taylor & Francis Group
Boca Raton London New York

CRC Press is an imprint of the
Taylor & Francis Group, an **informa** business

Designed cover: Shirley A. Bayer and Joseph Altman

First edition published 2024
by CRC Press
2385 NW Executive Center Drive, Suite 320, Boca Raton, FL 33431

and by CRC Press
4 Park Square, Milton Park, Abingdon, Oxon, OX14 4RN

CRC Press is an imprint of Taylor & Francis Group, LLC

LCCN no. 2022008216

ISBN: 978-1-032-22874-7 (hbk)
ISBN: 978-1-032-22004-8 (pbk)
ISBN: 978-1-003-27460-5 (ebk)

DOI: 10.1201/9781003274605

Typeset in Times Roman
by KnowledgeWorks Global Ltd.

Publisher's note: This book has been prepared from camera-ready copy provided by the authors.
Access the Support Material: www.routledge.com/9781032228747

CONTENTS

ACKNOWLEDGMENTS

We thank the late Dr. William DeMyer, pediatric neurologist at Indiana University Medical Center, for access to his personal library on human CNS development. We also thank the staff of the National Museum of Health and Medicine that were at the Armed Forces Institute of Pathology, Walter Reed Hospital, Washington, D.C. when we collected data in 1995 and 1996: Dr. Adrianne Noe, Director; Archibald J. Fobbs, Curator of the Yakovlev Collection; Elizabeth C. Lockett; and William Discher. We are most grateful to the late Dr. James M. Petras at the Walter Reed Institute of Research who made his darkroom facilities available so that we could develop all the photomicrographs on location rather than in our laboratory in Indiana. Finally, we thank Chuck Crumly, Neha Bhatt, Kara Roberts, Michele Dimont, and Rebecca Condit for expert help during production of the manuscript.

AUTHORS

Shirley A. Bayer received her PhD from Purdue University in 1974 and spent most of her scientific career working with Joseph Altman. She was a professor of biology at Indiana-Purdue University in Indianapolis for several years, where she taught courses in human anatomy and developmental neurobiology while continuing to do research in brain development. Her lengthy publication record of dozens of peer-reviewed, scientific journal articles extends back to the mid 1970s. She has co-authored several books and many articles with her late spouse, Joseph Altman. It was her research (published in *Science* in 1982) that proved that new neurons are added to granule cells in the dentate gyrus during adult life, a unique neuronal population that grows. That paper stimulated interest in the dormant field of adult neurogenesis.

Joseph Altman, now deceased, was born in Hungary and migrated with his family via Germany and Australia to the US. In New York, he became a graduate student in psychology in the laboratory of Hans-Lukas Teuber, earning a PhD in 1959 from New York University. He was a postdoctoral fellow at Columbia University, and later joined the faculty at the Massachusetts Institute of Technology. In 1968, he accepted a position as a professor of biology at Purdue University. During his career, he collaborated closely with Shirley A. Bayer. From the early 1960s-2016, he published many articles in peer-reviewed journals, books, monographs, and free online books that emphasized developmental processes in brain anatomy and function. His most important discovery was adult neurogenesis, the creation of new neurons in the adult brain. This discovery was made in the early 1960s while he was based at MIT, but was largely ignored in favor of the prevailing dogma that neurogenesis is limited to prenatal development. After Dr. Bayer's paper proved new neurons are added to granule cells in the hippocampus, Dr. Altman's monumental discovery became more accepted. During the 1990s, new researchers "rediscovered" and confirmed his original finding. Adult neurogenesis has recently been proven to occur in the dentate gyrus, olfactory bulb, and striatum through the measurement of Carbon-14—the levels of which changed during nuclear bomb testing throughout the 20th century—in postmortem human brains. Today, many laboratories around the world are continuing to study the importance of adult neurogenesis in brain function. In 2011, Dr. Altman was awarded the Prince of Asturias Award, an annual prize given in Spain by the Prince of Asturias Foundation to individuals, entities, or organizations globally who make notable achievements in the sciences, humanities, and public affairs. In 2012, he received the International Prize for Biology - an annual award from the Japan Society for the Promotion of Science (JSPS) for "outstanding contribution to the advancement of research in fundamental biology." This Prize is one of the most prestigious honors a scientist can receive. When Dr. Altman died in 2016, Dr. Bayer continued the work they started over 50 years ago. In her late husband's honor, she created the Altman Prize, awarded each year by JSPS to an outstanding young researcher in developmental neuroscience.

INTRODUCTION

A. Specimens and Organization

Volume 11 in this Atlas Series presents the human brain in two normal specimens from the Yakovlev Collection[1] at 6.5 months during the early third trimester. These specimens were analyzed in Volume 2 of the original *Atlas of Human Central Nervous System Development* (Bayer and Altman, 2004). By this time, most fetuses are viable *ex utero*. Nearly all the structures present in the adult brain are recognizable and are maturing from the diencephalon to the medulla. But remnants of the embryonic nervous system remain, mainly in the cerebral cortex and in the cerebellar cortex.

This volume contains serial grayscale photographs of Nissl-stained sections of a sagittal specimen (Y147-

1. The *Yakovlev Collection* (designated by a **Y** prefix in the specimen number) is the work of Dr. Paul Ivan Yakovlev (1894–1983), a neurologist affiliated with Harvard University. Throughout his career, Yakovlev collected many diseased and normal human brains. He invented a giant microtome that was capable of sectioning entire human brains. Later, he became interested in the developing brain and collected many during the second and third trimesters. The normal brains in the developmental group were cataloged by Haleem (1990) and were examined by us during 1996 and 1997. The collection was moved to the National Museum of Health and Medicine when the Armed Forces Institute of Pathology (AFIP) closed at Walter Reed Hospital and is still available for research.

63, **Part II**) and a horizontal specimen (Y16-59, **Part III**) with crown-rump (CR) lengths of 225 mm and 235 mm, respectively. Both specimens are approximately in the 26th gestational week (GW).

Sagittal Plates are ordered from medial to lateral; the anterior part of each photographed section is facing left, posterior right. **Horizontal Plates** are presented from dorsal (first) to ventral (last); the anterior part of each section faces left, the posterior part faces right; the midline is in the vertical center. Each **Plate** is in two parts: **A,** on the left, shows the full-contrast photograph without labels; **B,** on the right, shows a low-contrast copy of each photograph with unabbreviated labels. For each specimen, a series of serially spaced **low-magnification plates** show the entire section to identify large structures. The brain core is shown in many **high-magnification plates** to identify smaller structures. In addition, several **very-high-magnification plates** show the cerebral and cerebellar cortices. Because our emphasis is on development, transient structures that appear only in immature brains are labeled in ***italics***, either directly in some of the high-magnification plates or in **bold numbers** that refer to labels in a list. During dissection, embedding, cutting, and staining, some of the sections illustrated were torn; that damage is sometimes surrounded by *dashed lines*.

B. Developmental Highlights

Figures 1-2 compare second trimester and early third trimester brains in horizontal sections of the dorsal telencephalon. The overall growth of the brain is obvious when the sections are stacked in a "layer cake" arrangement (**Fig. 1**). The side-by-side comparison (**Fig. 2**) shows that parts of the cerebral cortex are growing at different rates. From GW 20 to GW 23 to GW 26, the cortical plate gradually increases its thickness and rapidly grows lengthwise. The white matter (*pale yellow*) greatly increases its thickness in most cortical areas except the insula. On the other hand, layers 3-6 of the *stratified transitional field* slow their growth, especially between GW 20 and GW 23; by GW 26, these layers have nearly disappeared in the frontal areas and are very thin in posterior (occipital) areas. Synchronously with these growth dynamics, the cortex begins to fold outward (gyri) and inward (sulci and fissures) to accommodate the rapidly increasing surface area.

Cortical gyrification is an intriguing phenomenon that neuroanatomists have studied for many years; Welker (1990) wrote a comprehensive review of the literature in mammals (including humans). The abstract of his review is that uneven expansion of cortical areas cause gyri and sulci to develop, with

Superimposed Early Third Trimester and Second Trimester Brains in the Horizontal Plane

Bottom layer: GW 26
Middle layer: GW 23
Top layer: GW 20

NEP- neuroepithelium
STF-stratified transitional field
SVZ-subventricular zone

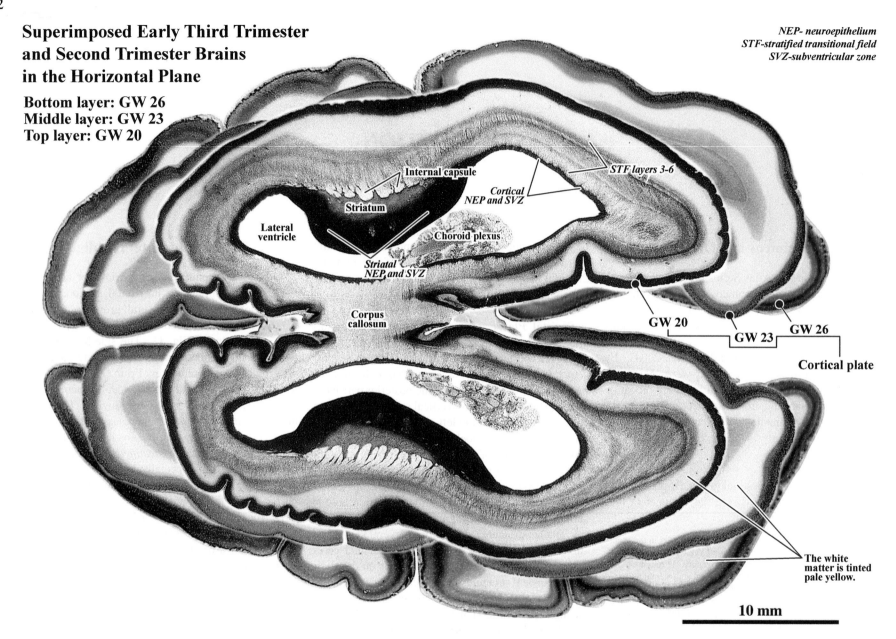

Figures 1 and 2 (*facing pages*). A comparison of second and early third trimester brains in the horizontal plane to show the relative growth of different components of the cerebral cortex. Note that the internal capsule and corpus callosum are well established by GW 20. Massive growth of fibers into the white matter (*pale yellow*) from subcortical areas (mainly the thalamus) and from neurons within the cortical plate growing axons into the white matter (some extend to the opposite side in the corpus callosum) are related to the formation of fissures, sulci, and gyri. (GW 20 is shown in Plate 41, Volume 9, Bayer and Altman, in Press; GW 23 in Plate 1, Volume 10, Bayer and Altman, in Press; GW 26 in Plate 28, this Volume).

Side-by-Side Comparison of Early Third Trimester and Second Trimester Brains in the Horizontal Plane

Growth related to increased gyrification:
Cortical plate increases thickness and linear surface
White matter increases depth in most areas (insula excepted)
STF layers 3-6 decrease in relative size

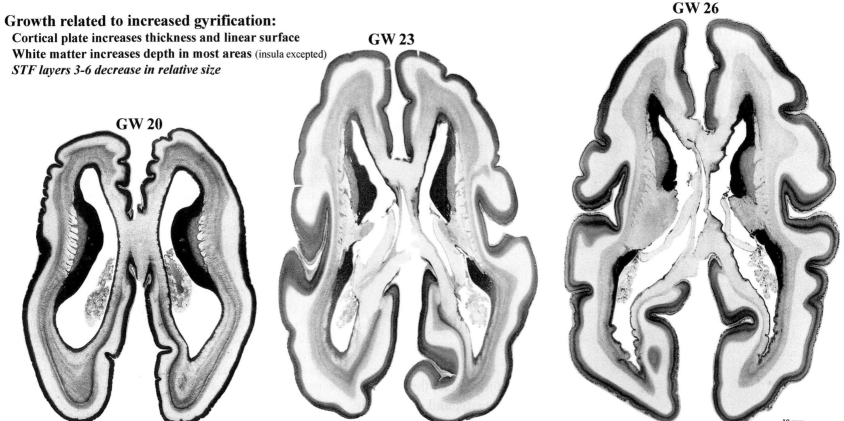

GW 26

GW 23

GW 20

10 mm

slower- growing parts of cortex in the fundus of a sulcus and faster-growing cortex in the walls and the crowns of a gyrus. Our observations concur that uneven growth results in gyrification and also puts forth the hypothesis that the pattern of cortical gyrification results from the establishment of early anatomical connections with specific areas of the cortical plate (Altman and Bayer, 2015). Our hypothesis is that early connections with the thalamus "anchor" specific areas of the cortical plate (*see* Fig. 2, Volume 10, Bayer and Altman, in press, also Van Essen, 1997) and initiates the process of gyrification. Thalamic

neurogenesis is completed during the middle part of the first trimester, and it is plausible that some early contacts are made that set off unique cortical areas. Furthermore, thalamic axons are a main component of the internal capsule fiber tract[2] that first appears on GW 8.4 (*see* Plates 20-21, Volume 4, Bayer and Altman, 2023)

2. The internal capsule is a major tract in the telencephalon that links the cortex to subcortical structures. Some of its components are afferent axons from the brainstem (e.g., locus coeruleus), thalamo-cortical axons, cortico-thalamic axons, axons that will form the corticospinal and corticobulbar tracts, and axons that run to and from the basal ganglia.

The first anchoring occurs with the ventrolateral cortical plate that will become the insula at the base of the lateral fissure. The insula divides the lateral cortex into an anterior frontal lobe and a posterior temporal lobe. The cortical plate appears first in the future insula on GW 8.4 (*see* Plates 19-20, Volume 4, Bayer and Altman, 2022). By GW 9.6, the cortical plate is extensive throughout the entire cerebral wall but is most thick in a central lateral area (insula) that has a slight indentation. This part of the cortex is directly adjacent to the entry zone of the massive internal capsule (*see* Plate 5, Volume 5, Bayer and Altman, 2023).

4

Anatomical Connections Contribute to the Establishment of the Lateral Fissure and Central Sulcus

Thalamic **ventral nuclear complexes (VA, VL, VPL, VPM)** project to primary motor cortex on the anterior bank and primary somatosensory cortex on the posterior bank of the **central sulcus**.

Thalamic nuclei that relay **smell, taste, and autonomic functions** project to the insular cortex at the base of the **lateral fissure**.

Figure 3. A lateral sagittal section of the brain of Y147-63 from **Plate 9** in **Part II** of this volume is used to indicate the anatomical connections of the sensorimotor cortex (*top*) around the central sulcus and some anatomical connections of the insula (*bottom*). Abbreviations: VA, ventral anterior nucleus (relays input from the globus pallidus); VL, ventral lateral nucleus (relays input from the cerebellum); VPL, ventral posterolateral nucleus (relays touch and pain from the medial lemniscus and the spinothalamic tracts from the lower limbs and trunk); VPM, ventral posteromedial nucleus (relays touch and pain from the medial lemniscus and the spinothalamic tracts from the upper limbs and trunk).

All parts of the mature insular cortex are contacted by thalamic nuclei, especially those related to olfaction, taste, and autonomic functions (**Fig. 3**, Ghaziri et al., 2018).

The next cortical area to be cordoned off is the primary visual cortex in the depths of the calcarine fissure (**Fig. 4**). On GW 14, a sharp and deep indent occurs in the posteriomedial cerebral wall (*see* Plates 10-13, Volume 8, Bayer and Altman, in press), the presumptive calcarine sulcus. Already by the end of the first trimester, some internal capsule fibers can be seen curving sharply back toward the posterior cortex (*see* Plates 5-6, Volume 7, Bayer and Altman, 2023). The lateral geniculate body in the thalamus gets point-to-point input from retinal ganglion cells and then relays that ordered input to both sides of the calcarine sulcus so that the lower visual field maps to the cuneus and the upper visual field maps to the lingula.

The parieto-occipital sulcus appears slightly later than the calcarine sulcus, and the two form an L-shaped cleft in the medial cortical wall in sagittal sections (**Fig. 4**). The anterior side of the sulcus (visual area 6) gets strong input from the large pulvinar nucleus in the thalamus that relays secondary visual information as well as other sensory modalities (Gamberini, et al. 2015). It is our hypothesis that initial connections with this part of the cortex contributes to the establishment of the sulcus and the posterior extent of the parietal lobe.

The paracentral lobule that surrounds both sides of the central sulcus (**Fig. 3**) appears first on GW 20 in the ventrolateral cortical plate (*see* Plates 15 and 36, Volume 9, Bayer and Altman, in press). That corresponds to our findings in rats (Bayer and Altman, 1991), now also in humans (the current Atlas Series), that ventrolateral cortical areas develop earlier than dorsomedial areas. The central sulcus is prominent in lateral sagittal sections (**Fig. 3**), and absent in medial sections (*compare* **Plates 4 and 10 in Part II** of this Volume). It is well known that the large ventral nuclear complexes in the thalamus project to the primary motor area on the anterior bank of the central sulcus (for a review and a recent current study, *see* Rouiller, et al., 1999), and the same thalamic areas also project to the primary somatosensory cortex on the posterior bank of the sulcus (Huffman and Krubitzer, 2001). These projections are topographically organized and produce a map of the body parts (the homunculus) on both primary motor and primary somatosensory cortices. There is a homunculus in rats as well, and we found that the pattern of anatomical connections with the thalamus can be linked to the neurogenetic gradients in both the thalamus and the cortex (Bayer and Altman, 1991).

By the beginning of the third trimester, all major gyri and sulci have appeared and the vast cortical sheet is presumably shaped by early connections with the thalamus. The result is seven anatomical areas.

First, the limbic lobe ("edge" lobe) was not discussed, but much of it is established by GW 7.4 as the hippocampus becomes definite in the dorsomedial edge of the cerebral cortex adjacent to the presumptive cingulate cortex (see Plates 24-25, Volume 3, Bayer and Altman 2023). That is before the cortical plate appears and is due to intrinsic gene expression of the LIM-homeodomain gene *Lhx2* (Bulchand et al., 2001). Growth of the entire cortex causes the ventral hippocampus and the parahippocampal cortex to be displaced near the insula (*see* Plates 10 and 11, Volume 6, Bayer and Altman, 2023). **Second and third**, the lateral frontal and the temporal lobes are established by the end of the first trimester. They grow backward and forward respectively to cover the insula during the second trimester. **Fourth**, the primary visual cortex and secondary visual cortex in the occipital lobe around the calcarine and parieto-occipital sulci appear in the early second trimester. **Fifth**, the paracentral lobule surrounding the central sulcus also appears in the second trimester ventrolaterally and gradually extends dorsomedially during the third trimester. **Sixth**, the medial frontal lobe anterior to the precentral gyrus is cordoned off in the late second trimester. **Seventh**, the medial parietal lobe posterior to the postcentral gyrus is cordoned off in the late second trimester. Secondary and tertiary gyrification will continue through the third trimester, after birth, into infancy, childhood, juvenile ages, and not come to an end until the young adult period.

Anatomical Connections Contribute to the Establishment of the Calcarine and Parieto-occipital Sulci

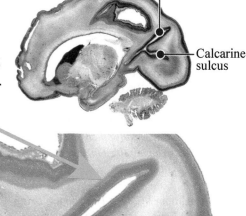

The thalamic **pulvinar** projects to area V6 on the anterior bank of the **parieto-occipital sulcus**.

The thalamic **lateral geniculate body** projects to the primary visual cortex on opposite sides of the **calcarine sulcus**.

LOWER VISUAL FIELD
UPPER VISUAL FIELD

Cuneus

Lingula

10 mm

Figure 4. A midlateral sagittal section of the brain of Y147-63 from **Plate 5 in Part II** of this volume is used to indicate the anatomical connections surrounding the parieto-occipital sulcus (*top orange arrow*) and the point-to-point input of the primary visual cortex surrounding the calcarine sulcus (*bottom pink and green arrows*). The upper visual field in the lingula maps the individual's world-centered space, while the lower visual field in the cuneus maps the individual's egocentric space. Visual association cortex around the parieto-occipital sulcus contains areas involved with eye-hand coordination during reaching and grasping (*see* Figure 77 in Altman and Bayer, 2015). Note that the central sulcus is less deep here than in the section in **Figure 3**.

6

REFERENCES

Altman J, Bayer SA. (2015) *Development of the Human Neocortex.* Ocala, FL, Laboratory of Developmental Neurobiology, neurondevelopment.org.

Bayer SA, Altman J (1991) *Neocortical Development.* New York: Raven Press.

Bayer SA, Altman J (2004) *Atlas of Human Central Nervous System Development*, Volume 2: *The Human Bran during the Third Trimester.* Boca Raton, FL, CRC Press.

Bayer SA, Altman J (2023) *The Human Brain during the First Trimester 15- to 18-mm Crown-Rump Lengths, Atlas of Human Central Nervous System Development*, Volume 3. Taylor and Francis, CRC Press.

Bayer SA, Altman J (2023) *The Human Brain during the First Trimester 21- to 23-mm Crown-Rump Lengths, Atlas of Human Central Nervous System Development*, Volume 4. Taylor and Francis, CRC Press.

Bayer SA, Altman J (2023) *The Human Brain during the First Trimester 31- to 33-mm Crown-Rump Lengths, Atlas of Human Central Nervous System Development*, Volume 5. Taylor and Francis, CRC Press.

Bayer SA, Altman J (2023) *The Human Brain during the First Trimester 40- to 42-mm Crown-Rump Lengths, Atlas of Human Central Nervous System Development*, Volume 6. Taylor and Francis, CRC Press.

Bayer SA, Altman J (2023) *The Human Brain during the First Trimester 57- to 60-mm Crown-Rump Lengths, Atlas of Human Central Nervous System Development*, Volume 7. Taylor and Francis, CRC Press.

Bayer SA, Altman J (2023) *The Human Brain during the Second Trimester 96- to 150-mm Crown-Rump Lengths, Atlas of Human Central Nervous System Development*, Volume 8. Taylor and Francis, CRC Press.

Bayer SA, Altman J (in press) *The Human Brain during the Second Trimester 160- to 170-mm Crown-Rump Lengths, Atlas of Human Central Nervous System Development*, Volume 9. Taylor and Francis, CRC Press.

Bayer SA, Altman J (in press) *The Human Brain during the Second Trimester 190- to 210-mm Crown-Rump Lengths, Atlas of Human Central Nervous System Development*, Volume 10. Taylor and Francis, CRC Press.

Bulchand S, Grove EA, Porter JD Tole S. (2001) LIM-homeodomain gene *Lhx2* regulates the formation of the cortical hem. *Mechanisms of Development*, 100:165-175.

Curtis BA, Jacobson S, Marcus EM (1972) *An Introduction to the Neurosciences*, Philadelphia: W. B. Saunders.

Gamberini M, Bakola S, Passarelli L, et al. (2015) Thalamic projections to visual and visuomotor areas (V6 and V6a in the rostral bank of the parieto-occipital sulcus of the macaque. *Brain Structure and Function* 221:1573-1589

Ghaziri J, Tucholka A, Girard G, et al. (2018) Subcortical structural connectivity of insular subregions. *Scientific Reports* 8:8596, www.nature.com/scientificreports

Haleem M (1990) *Diagnostic Categories of the Yakovlev Collection of Normal and Pathological Anatomy and Development of the Brain.* Washington, D.C. Armed Forces Institute of Pathology.

Huffman KJ, Krubitzer L (2001) Thalamo-cortical connections of areas 3a and M1 in marmoset monkeys. *Journal of Comparative Neurology* 435:291-310.

Larroche JC (1966) The development of the central nervous system during intrauterine life. In: *Human Development*, F. Falkner (ed.), Philadelphia: W. B. Saunders, pages 257-276.

Rouiller EM, Tanne J, Moret V, Boussaoud D (1999) Origin of thalamic inputs to the primary, premotor, and supplementary motor cortical areas and to area 46 in macaque monkeys: a multiple retrograde tracing study. *Journal of Comparative Neurology*, 409:131-152.

Van Essen DC (1997) A tension-based theory of morphogenesis and compact wiring in the central nervous system. *Nature*, 385:313-318.

Welker W. (1990) Why does the cerebral cortex fissure and fold? A review of determinants of gyri and sulci. In: *Cerebral Cortex*, Jones E G et al., eds. New York: Springer Science and Business Media, pages 3-136.

PART II: Y147-63
CR 225 mm (GW 26)
Sagittal

This specimen is case number W-147-63 (Perinatal RPSL) in the Yakovlev Collection. A female infant survived for 27 days after a premature birth. Death occurred from a hemorrhage in the abdominal cavity. The brain was cut in the sagittal plane in 35-μm thick sections and is classified as a Normative Control in the Yakovlev Collection (Haleem, 1990). Since there is no photograph of this brain before it was embedded and cut, the photograph of the medial view of a GW 25 brain that Larroche published in 1966 (**Figure 5**) is used to show gross anatomical features.

Photographs of 10 different Nissl-stained sections are shown in full in **Plates 1-10**. High-magnification views of the brain core and cerebellum are featured in **Plates 11-20**. Very-high-magnification views of different regions of the cerebellar cortex are shown in **Plates 21-26**. Because the section numbers decrease from **Plate 1** (most medial) to **Plate 10** (most lateral), they are from the left side of the brain; the right side has higher section numbers proceeding medial to lateral. The cutting plane of this brain is nearly parallel to the midline in anterior and posterior parts of each section, including different parts of the cortex. The sections chosen for illustration are spaced closer together near the midline to show small structures in the diencephalon, midbrain, pons, and medulla.

Y147-63 contains several immature structures. In the telencephalon, remnants of the germinal zones are present in all lobes of the cerebral cortex where the **neuroepithelium/subventricular zone** is generating neocortical neurons. Migrating and sojourning neurons and/or glia are visible in all lobes of the cerebral cortex in **stratified transitional fields**, thin but with prominent layering in the occipital lobe, and thicker with faint layering in the frontal, parietal, and temporal lobes. More neurons, glia, and their mitotic precursor cells are migrating through the olfactory peduncle toward the olfactory bulb (**rostral migratory stream**) from a presumed source area in the germinal matrix at the junction between the cerebral cortex, striatum, and nucleus accumbens. Streams of neurons and glia percolate through the claustrum, endopiriform nucleus, external capsule, and uncinate fasciculus in the **lateral migratory stream**. These cells appear to be heading toward the insular cortex, primary olfactory cortex, temporal cortex, and basolateral parts of the amygdaloid complex. In the basal ganglia, there is a thick **neuroepithelium/subventricular zone** overlying the striatum and nucleus accumbens where neurons and glia are being generated; some of these, especially from the accumbal area, will enter the **rostral migratory stream**. Another region of active neurogenesis in the telencephalon is the **subgranular zone** in the hilus

of the dentate gyrus that is the source of granule cells. The septum, fornix, and Ammon's horn have only a thin, darkly staining layer at the ventricle, and these are presumed to be generating glia, cells of the choroid plexus, and the ependymal lining of the ventricle.

Most of the structures in the diencephalon appear to be settled and are maturing, but the **glioepithelium/ependyma** lining the third ventricle is more thick than in the older specimens. A convoluted **glioepithelium/ependyma** lines the cerebral aqueduct in the midbrain. A smooth **glioepithelium/ependyma** lines the fourth ventricle through much of the pons. Another convoluted **glioepithelium/ependyma** lines the fourth ventricle through much of the medulla; part of that may be a remnant of the germinal source of the precerebellar nuclei. The **external germinal layer** is prominent over the entire surface of the cerebellar cortex and is actively producing basket, stellate, and granule cells. The **germinal trigone** is visible at the base of the nodulus and along the floccular peduncle; choroid plexus cells and glia are originating here and some migrating neurons may still be in the trigone.

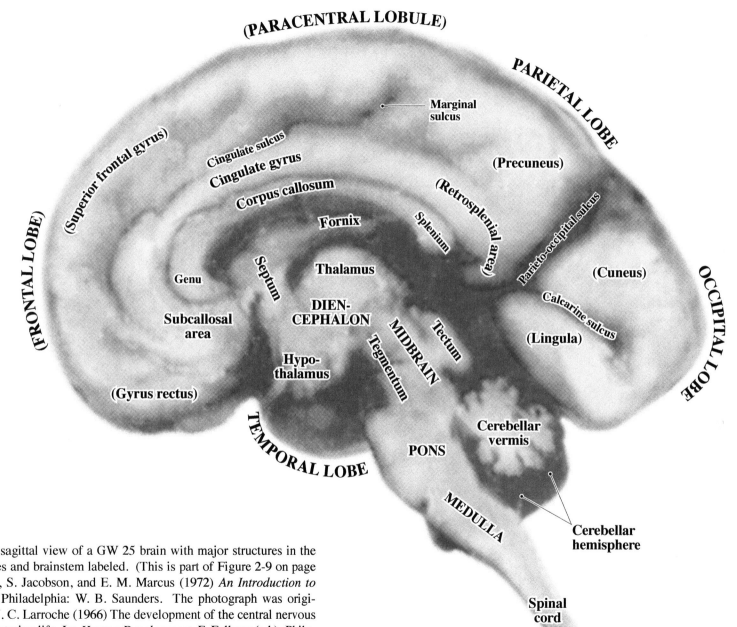

(PARACENTRAL LOBULE)

PARIETAL LOBE

Marginal
sulcus

Cingulate sulcus

Cingulate gyrus

(Superior frontal gyrus)

Corpus callosum

(Precuneus)

(Retrosplenial area)

Parieto-occipital sulcus

Fornix

Splenium

(FRONTAL LOBE)

OCCIPITAL LOBE

Thalamus

(Cuneus)

Genu

Septum

**DIEN-
CEPHALON**

Calcarine sulcus

Subcallosal
area

MIDBRAIN

Tectum

(Lingula)

Hypo-
thalamus

Tegmentum

(Gyrus rectus)

Cerebellar
vermis

TEMPORAL LOBE

PONS

MEDULLA

Cerebellar
hemisphere

Spinal
cord

Figure 5. Midline sagittal view of a GW 25 brain with major structures in the cerebral hemispheres and brainstem labeled. (This is part of Figure 2-9 on page 27 in B. A. Curtis, S. Jacobson, and E. M. Marcus (1972) *An Introduction to the Neurosciences*, Philadelphia: W. B. Saunders. The photograph was originally published by J. C. Larroche (1966) The development of the central nervous system during intrauterine life. In: *Human Development*, F. Falkner (ed.), Philadelphia: W. B. Saunders, page 259.)

PLATE 1A
CR 225 mm
GW 26, Y147-63
Sagittal
Section 501

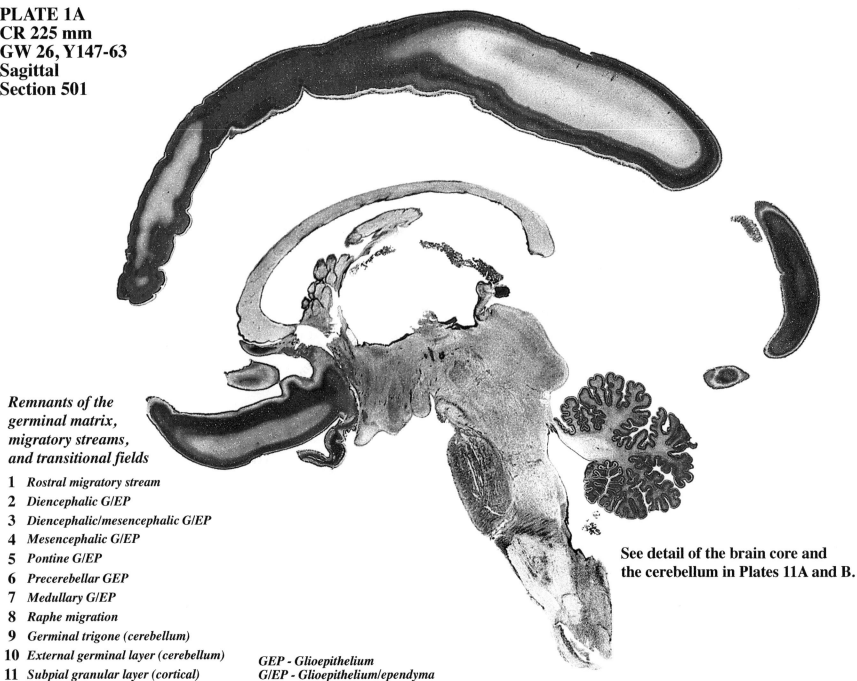

Remnants of the
germinal matrix,
migratory streams,
and transitional fields

1   *Rostral migratory stream*
2   *Diencephalic G/EP*
3   *Diencephalic/mesencephalic G/EP*
4   *Mesencephalic G/EP*
5   *Pontine G/EP*
6   *Precerebellar GEP*
7   *Medullary G/EP*
8   *Raphe migration*
9   *Germinal trigone (cerebellum)*
10 *External germinal layer (cerebellum)*
11 *Subpial granular layer (cortical)*

GEP - Glioepithelium
G/EP - Glioepithelium/ependyma

See detail of the brain core and
the cerebellum in Plates 11A and B.

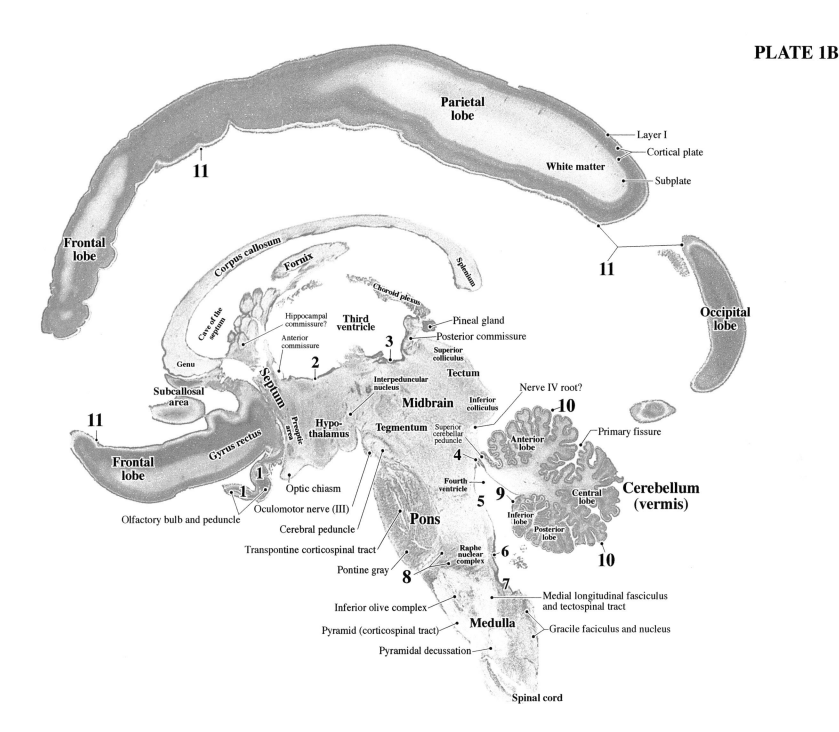

Parietal lobe

Layer I
Cortical plate
White matter
Subplate

Frontal lobe

Corpus callosum
Fornix
Splenium

11

11

Occipital lobe

Cave of the septum
Hippocampal commissure?
Third ventricle
Choroid plexus
Pineal gland
Posterior commissure

Anterior commissure

Genu

Septum
3
Superior colliculus
Tectum

Interpeduncular nucleus

2

Subcallosal area

Nerve IV root?

10

Midbrain
Inferior colliculus

Hypo-thalamus

Preoptic area

Tegmentum
Superior cerebellar peduncle

Anterior lobe

Primary fissure

11

Gyrus rectus

4

Frontal lobe

1

Fourth ventricle

Central lobe

Cerebellum (vermis)

1

5
9

Optic chiasm

Inferior lobe

Posterior lobe

1

Oculomotor nerve (III)

Pons

Raphe nuclear complex

6

10

Olfactory bulb and peduncle

Cerebral peduncle

8

Transpontine corticospinal tract

Pontine gray

7

Medial longitudinal fasciculus and tectospinal tract

Inferior olive complex

Medulla

Pyramid (corticospinal tract)

Gracile faciculus and nucleus

Pyramidal decussation

Spinal cord

PLATE 2A
CR 225 mm
GW 26, Y147-63
Sagittal
Section 481

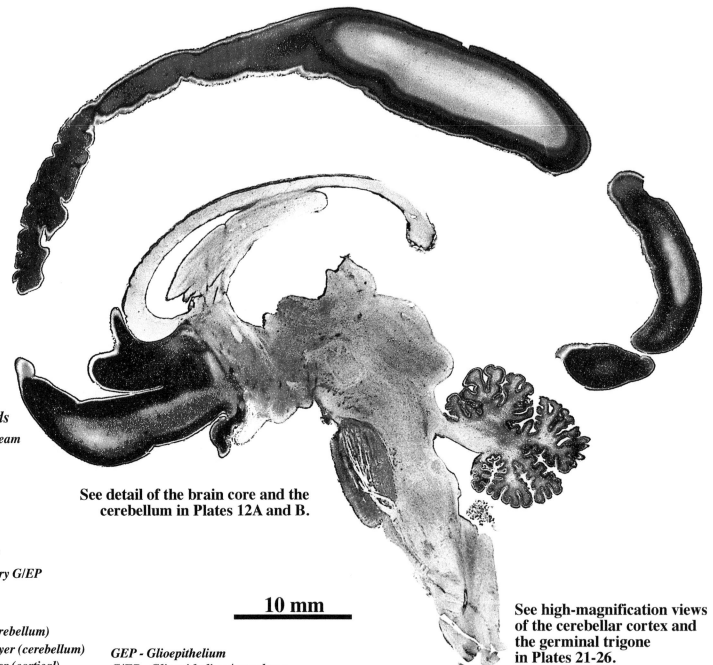

Remnants of the
germinal matrix,
migratory streams,
and transitional fields

1 *Rostral migratory stream*
2 *Callosal sling*
3 *Callosal GEP*
4 *Fornical GEP*
5 *Strionuclear GEP*
6 *Thalamic G/EP*
7 *Mesencephalic G/EP*
8 *Pontine and medullary G/EP*
9 *Raphe migration*
10 *Spinal G/EP*
11 *Germinal trigone (cerebellum)*
12 *External germinal layer (cerebellum)*
13 *Subpial granular layer (cortical)*

See detail of the brain core and the
cerebellum in Plates 12A and B.

10 mm

GEP - Glioepithelium
G/EP - Glioepithelium/ependyma

See high-magnification views
of the cerebellar cortex and
the germinal trigone
in Plates 21-26.

13

PLATE 2B

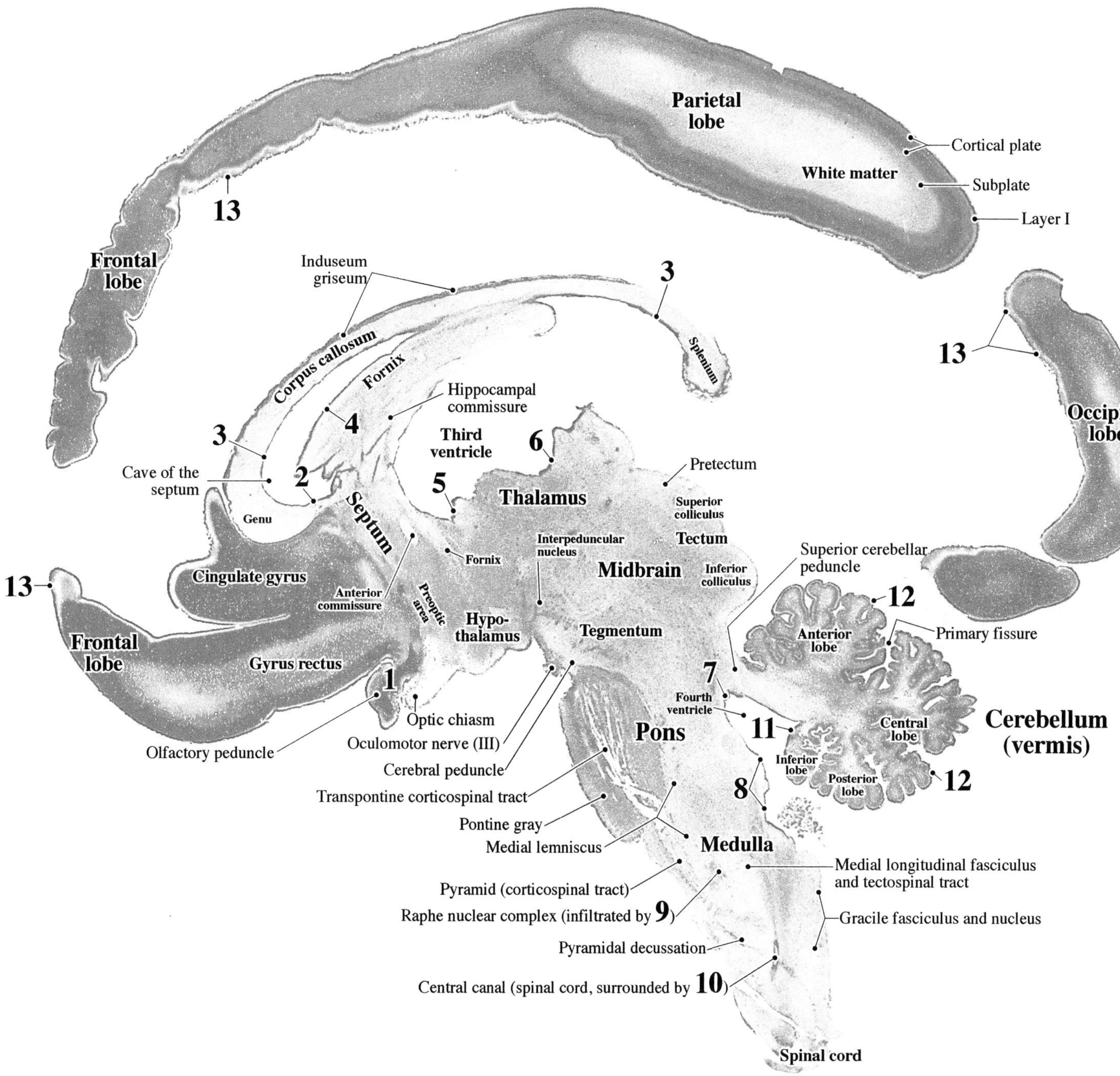

Parietal lobe

Cortical plate

White matter

Subplate

Layer I

Frontal lobe

13

Induseum griseum

3

Splenium

Occipital lobe

13

Corpus callosum

Fornix

Hippocampal commissure

Third ventricle

3

6

Pretectum

Cave of the septum

2

Septum

5

Thalamus

Superior colliculus

Tectum

Genu

Fornix

Interpeduncular nucleus

Midbrain

Inferior colliculus

Superior cerebellar peduncle

Cingulate gyrus

Anterior commissure

Preoptic area

Hypo-thalamus

Tegmentum

Primary fissure

Anterior lobe

12

13

Frontal lobe

1

7

Central lobe

Cerebellum (vermis)

Gyrus rectus

Optic chiasm

Oculomotor nerve (III)

Fourth ventricle

11

Inferior lobe

Olfactory peduncle

Cerebral peduncle

Pons

8

Posterior lobe

12

Transpontine corticospinal tract

Pontine gray

Medial lemniscus

Medulla

Medial longitudinal fasciculus and tectospinal tract

Pyramid (corticospinal tract)

Raphe nuclear complex (infiltrated by 9)

Gracile fasciculus and nucleus

Pyramidal decussation

Central canal (spinal cord, surrounded by 10)

Spinal cord

14

PLATE 3A
CR 225 mm
GW 26, Y147-63
Sagittal
Section 461

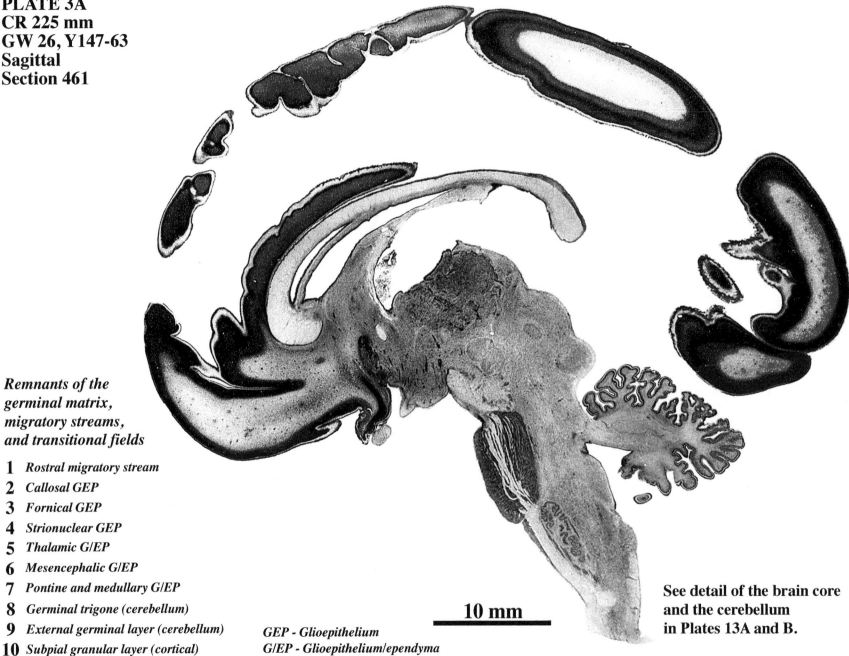

Remnants of the
germinal matrix,
migratory streams,
and transitional fields

1 *Rostral migratory stream*
2 *Callosal GEP*
3 *Fornical GEP*
4 *Strionuclear GEP*
5 *Thalamic G/EP*
6 *Mesencephalic G/EP*
7 *Pontine and medullary G/EP*
8 *Germinal trigone (cerebellum)*
9 *External germinal layer (cerebellum)*
10 *Subpial granular layer (cortical)*

10 mm

GEP - Glioepithelium
G/EP - Glioepithelium/ependyma

See detail of the brain core
and the cerebellum
in Plates 13A and B.

15

PLATE 3B

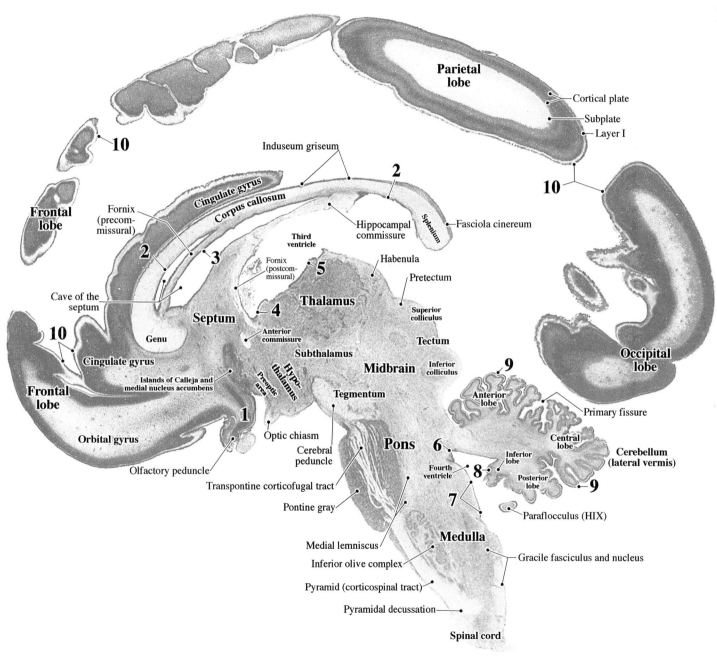

Parietal lobe

Cortical plate
Subplate
Layer I

10

Induseum griseum

2

Frontal lobe

10

Cingulate gyrus
Corpus callosum

Fornix (precommissural)

2

Hippocampal commissure

Splenium

Fasciola cinereum

Third ventricle

Fornix (postcommissural)

3

Habenula

Pretectum

5

Cave of the septum

Septum

4

Thalamus

Superior colliculus

Genu

Anterior commissure

Subthalamus

Tectum

10

Cingulate gyrus

Islands of Calleja and medial nucleus accumbens

Preoptic area

Hypo-thalamus

Midbrain

Inferior colliculus

Occipital lobe

9

Anterior lobe

Frontal lobe

Tegmentum

Primary fissure

Orbital gyrus

1

Optic chiasm

Pons

6

Central lobe

Olfactory peduncle

Cerebral peduncle

Inferior lobe

Cerebellum (lateral vermis)

Fourth ventricle

8

Posterior lobe

Transpontine corticofugal tract

7

9

Pontine gray

Paraflocculus (HIX)

Medial lemniscus

Medulla

Inferior olive complex

Gracile fasciculus and nucleus

Pyramid (corticospinal tract)

Pyramidal decussation

Spinal cord

16

PLATE 4A
CR 225 mm
GW 26, Y147-63
Sagittal
Section 421

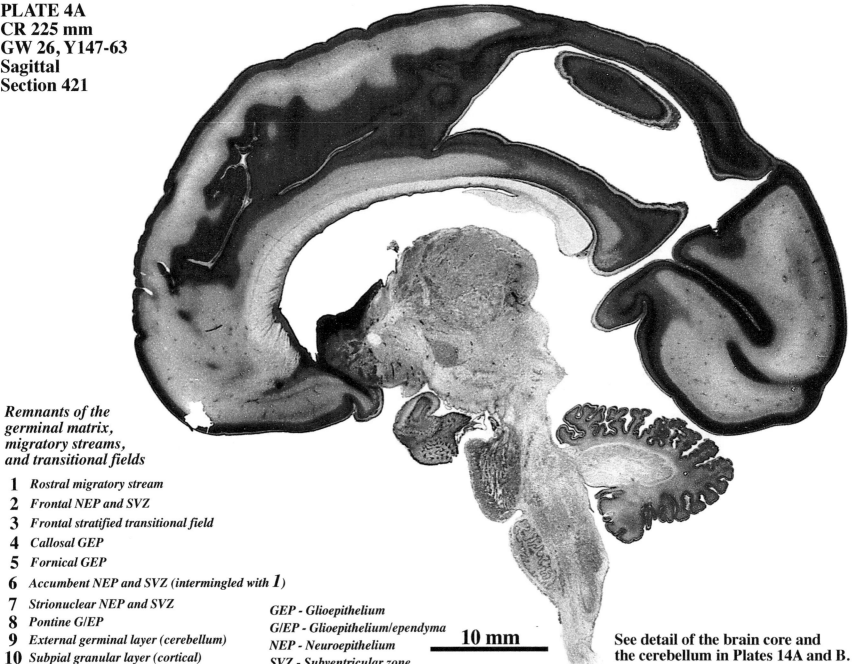

Remnants of the
germinal matrix,
migratory streams,
and transitional fields

1 *Rostral migratory stream*

2 *Frontal NEP and SVZ*

3 *Frontal stratified transitional field*

4 *Callosal GEP*

5 *Fornical GEP*

6 *Accumbent NEP and SVZ (intermingled with **1**)*

7 *Strionuclear NEP and SVZ*

8 *Pontine G/EP*

9 *External germinal layer (cerebellum)*

10 *Subpial granular layer (cortical)*

GEP - Glioepithelium
G/EP - Glioepithelium/ependyma
NEP - Neuroepithelium
SVZ - Subventricular zone

10 mm

See detail of the brain core and
the cerebellum in Plates 14A and B.

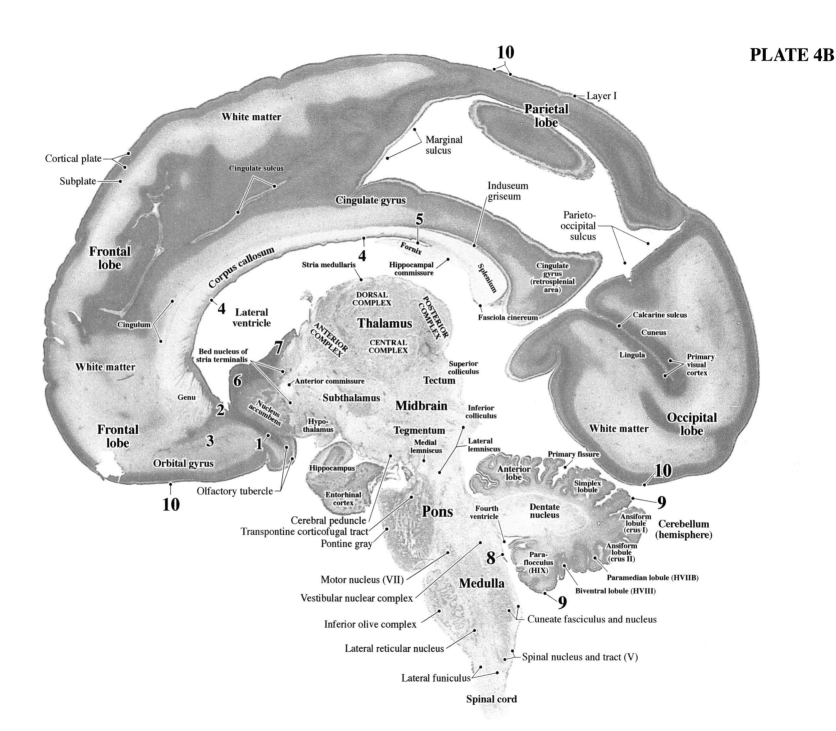

10

Layer I

Parietal lobe

White matter

Marginal sulcus

Cortical plate

Subplate

Cingulate sulcus

Induseum griseum

Parieto-occipital sulcus

Cingulate gyrus

5

Fornix

Frontal lobe

Corpus callosum

4

Stria medullaris

Hippocampal commissure

Splenium

Cingulate gyrus (retrosplenial area)

Fasciola cinereum

4 Lateral ventricle

Cingulum

DORSAL COMPLEX

POSTERIOR COMPLEX

Thalamus

Calcarine sulcus

Cuneus

ANTERIOR COMPLEX

CENTRAL COMPLEX

Lingula

Primary visual cortex

7

Bed nucleus of stria terminalis

6

Anterior commissure

Superior colliculus

Tectum

White matter

Genu

2

Nucleus accumbens

Subthalamus

Midbrain

Inferior colliculus

Occipital lobe

Frontal lobe

Hypo-thalamus

Tegmentum

Medial lemniscus

Lateral lemniscus

3

1

Primary fissure

10

Orbital gyrus

Hippocampus

Anterior lobe

Simplex lobule

9

Olfactory tubercle

Entorhinal cortex

Pons

Fourth ventricle

Dentate nucleus

Ansiform lobule (crus I)

Cerebellum (hemisphere)

10

Cerebral peduncle

Transpontine corticofugal tract

Pontine gray

8

Para-flocculus (HIX)

Ansiform lobule (crus II)

Paramedian lobule (HVIIB)

Motor nucleus (VII)

Medulla

Biventral lobule (HVIII)

Vestibular nuclear complex

9

Inferior olive complex

Cuneate fasciculus and nucleus

Lateral reticular nucleus

Spinal nucleus and tract (V)

Lateral funiculus

Spinal cord

PLATE 5A
CR 225 mm
GW 26, Y147-63
Sagittal
Section 381

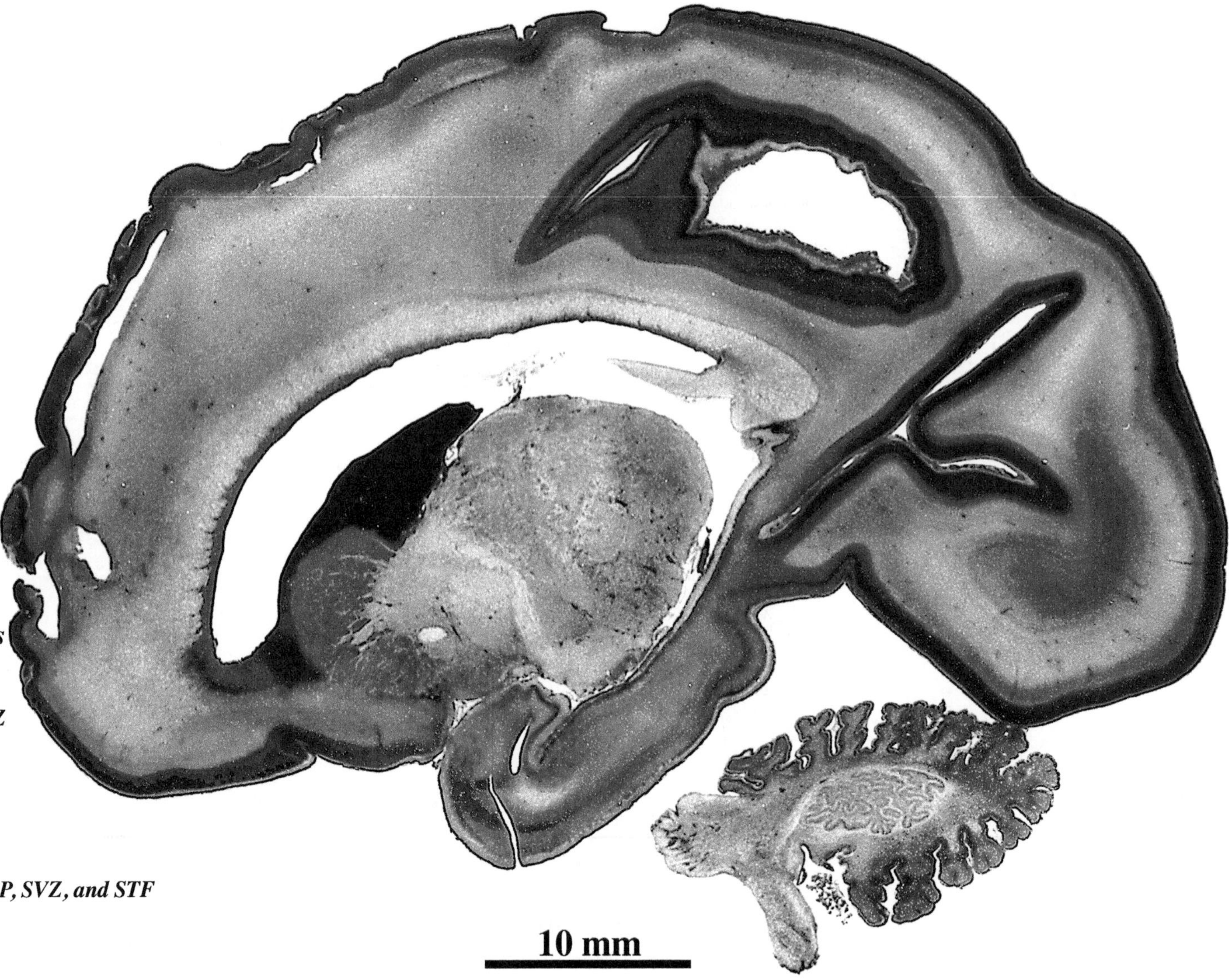

Remnants of the
germinal matrix,
migratory streams,
and transitional fields

1 *Rostral migratory*
   stream (source area)
2 *Frontal NEP and SVZ*
3 *Frontal STF*
4 *Callosal GEP*
5 *Fornical GEP*
6 *Occipital STF*
7 *Parahippocampal NEP, SVZ, and STF*
8 *Alvear GEP*
9 *Amygdaloid GE/P*
10 *Anterolateral striatal NEP and SVZ*
11 *Anteromedial striatal NEP and SVZ*
12 *Strionuclear GEP*
13 *External germinal layer (cerebellum)*
14 *Subpial granular layer (cortical)*

GEP - Glioepithelium
G/EP - Glioepithelium/ependyma
NEP - Neuroepithelium
STF - Stratified transitional field
SVZ - Subventricular zone

10 mm

See detail of the brain core and
the cerebellum in Plates 15A and B.

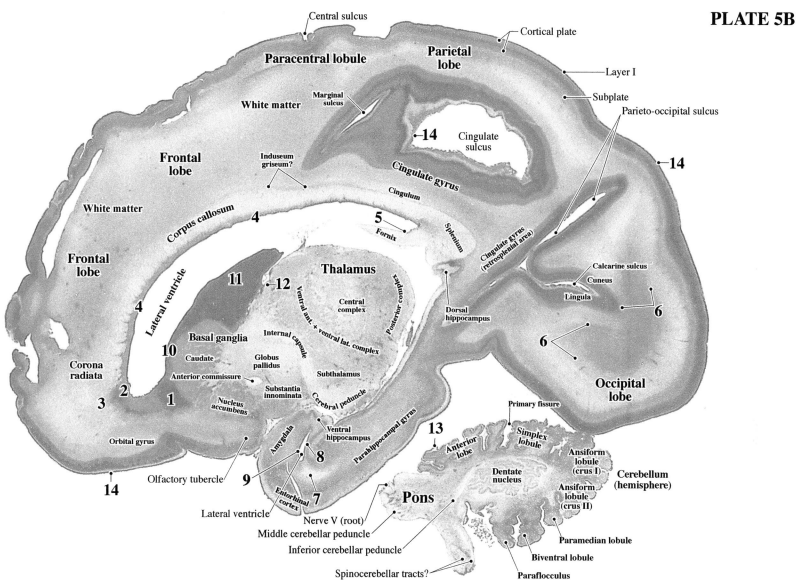

Central sulcus

Cortical plate

Paracentral lobule

Parietal lobe

Layer I

White matter

Marginal sulcus

Subplate

Parieto-occipital sulcus

Cingulate sulcus

-14

Frontal lobe

Induseum griseum?

Cingulate gyrus

-14

Cingulum

White matter

Corpus callosum

4

5

Splenium

Fornix

Cingulate gyrus (retrosplenial area)

Frontal lobe

Thalamus

Calcarine sulcus

11

-12

Ventral ant. + ventral lat. complex

Posterior complex

Cuneus

Central complex

Dorsal hippocampus

Lingula

6

Lateral ventricle

4

Internal capsule

Basal ganglia

6

Corona radiata

10

Caudate

Globus pallidus

Occipital lobe

Anterior commissure

Subthalamus

2

Substantia innominata

Cerebral peduncle

3

1

Nucleus accumbens

Primary fissure

13

Ventral hippocampus

Parahippocampal gyrus

Anterior lobe

Simplex lobule

Orbital gyrus

Amygdala

8

Ansiform lobule (crus I)

Cerebellum (hemisphere)

9

Dentate nucleus

Ansiform lobule (crus II)

14

Olfactory tubercle

Entorhinal cortex

7

Pons

Lateral ventricle

Nerve V (root)

Middle cerebellar peduncle

Paramedian lobule

Inferior cerebellar peduncle

Biventral lobule

Spinocerebellar tracts?

Paraflocculus

PLATE 6A
CR 225 mm
GW 26, Y147-63
Sagittal
Section 361

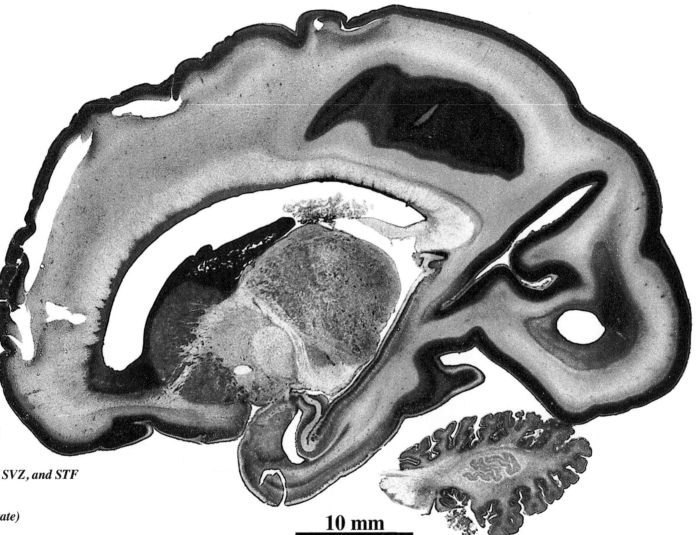

Remnants of the
germinal matrix,
migratory streams,
and transitional fields

1 *Rostral migratory*
  stream (source area)
2 *Frontal NEP and SVZ*
3 *Frontal STF*
4 *Callosal GEP*
5 *Fornical GEP*
6 *Occipital NEP and SVZ*
7 *Occipital STF*
8 *Parahippocampal NEP, SVZ, and STF*
9 *Alvear GEP*
10 *Subgranular zone (dentate)*
11 *Amygdaloid G/EP*
12 *Anterolateral striatal NEP and SVZ*
13 *Anteromedial striatal NEP and SVZ*
14 *Strionuclear GEP*
15 *External germinal layer (cerebellum)*
16 *Subpial granular layer (cortical)*

10 mm

GEP - Glioepithelium
G/EP - Glioepithelium/ependyma
NEP - Neuroepithelium
STF - Stratified transitional field
SVZ - Subventricular zone

See detail of the brain core and
the cerebellum in Plates 16A and B.

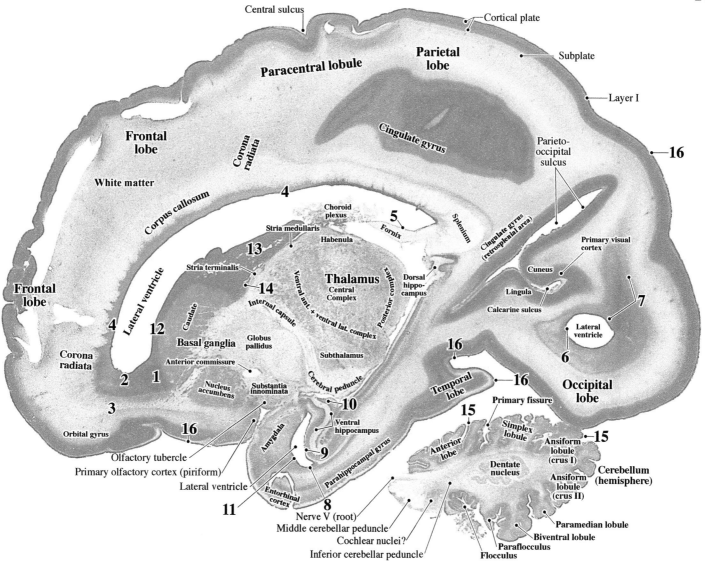

Central sulcus

Cortical plate

Parietal lobe

Paracentral lobule

Subplate

Layer I

Frontal lobe

Corona radiata

Cingulate gyrus

Parieto-occipital sulcus

16

White matter

Corpus callosum

4

Choroid plexus

5

Splenium

Cingulate gyrus (retrosplenial area)

Stria medullaris

Fornix

Primary visual cortex

13

Habenula

Cuneus

Lateral ventricle

Stria terminalis

Thalamus

Central Complex

Dorsal hippo-campus

Lingula

14

Ventral ant. + ventral lat. complex

Posterior complex

Calcarine sulcus

7

Frontal lobe

Caudate

Internal capsule

4 Lateral ventricle **12**

Basal ganglia

Globus pallidus

Lateral ventricle

6

Corona radiata

2 **1**

Anterior commissure

Subthalamus

16

16

7

Cerebral peduncle

Nucleus accumbens

Substantia innominata

Cerebral peduncle

Temporal lobe

16

Occipital lobe

3

Amygdala

10

Ventral hippocampus

Primary fissure

15

Simplex lobule

Ansiform lobule (crus I)

15

Orbital gyrus

16

9

Anterior lobe

Olfactory tubercle

Parahippocampal gyrus

Dentate nucleus

Cerebellum (hemisphere)

Primary olfactory cortex (piriform)

Lateral ventricle

Entorhinal cortex

Ansiform lobule (crus II)

11

8

Nerve V (root)

Middle cerebellar peduncle

Cochlear nuclei?

Inferior cerebellar peduncle

Paraflocculus

Flocculus

Paramedian lobule

Biventral lobule

PLATE 7A
CR 225 mm
GW 26, Y147-63
Sagittal
Section 341

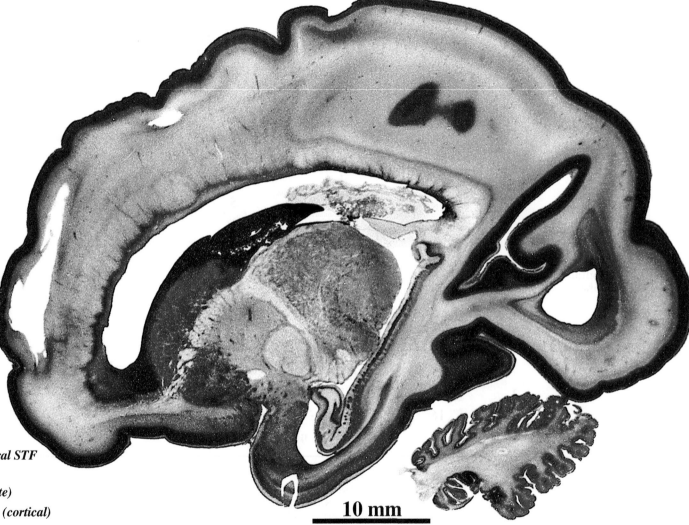

*Remnants of the
germinal matrix,
migratory streams,
and transitional fields*

1 *Rostral migratory
stream (source area)*

2 *Frontal NEP and SVZ*

3 *Frontal STF*

4 *Callosal GEP*

5 *Fornical GEP*

6 *Occipital NEP and SVZ*

7 *Occipital STF*

8 *Temporal NEP and SVZ*

9 *Parahippocampal/temporal STF*

10 *Alvear GEP*

11 *Subgranular zone (dentate)*

12 *Lateral migratory stream (cortical)*

13 *Amygdaloid G/EP*

14 *Anterolateral striatal NEP and SVZ*

15 *Anteromedial striatal NEP and SVZ*

16 *Strionuclear GEP*

17 *External germinal layer (cerebellum)*

18 *Subpial granular layer (cortical)*

10 mm

GEP - *Glioepithelium*
G/EP - *Glioepithelium/ependyma*
NEP - *Neuroepithelium*
STF - *Stratified transitional field*
SVZ - *Subventricular zone*

**See detail of the brain core and
the cerebellum in Plates 17A and B.**

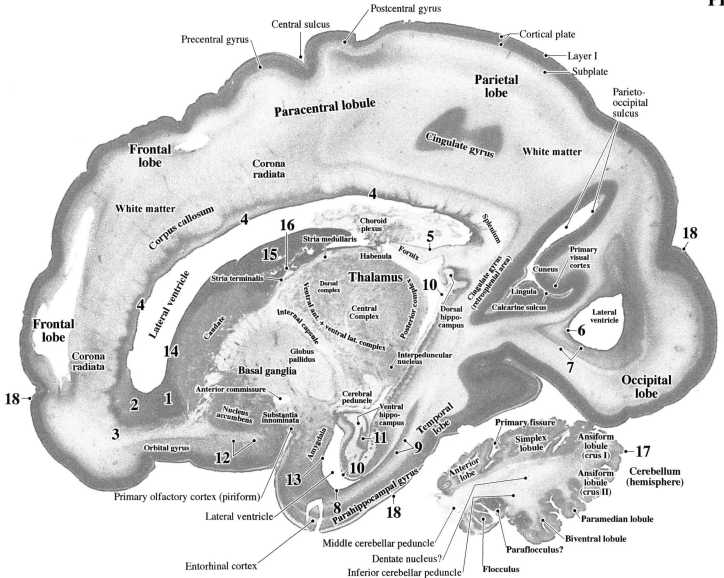

Precentral gyrus

Central sulcus

Postcentral gyrus

Cortical plate

Layer I

Subplate

Parietal lobe

Parieto-occipital sulcus

Paracentral lobule

Frontal lobe

Corona radiata

Cingulate gyrus

White matter

White matter

Corpus callosum

4

Choroid plexus

Splenium

18

16

Stria medullaris

5

Primary visual cortex

15

Habenula

Fornix

4

Cuneus

Stria terminalis

Dorsal complex

Thalamus

Cingulate gyrus (retrosplenial area)

Lingula

Lateral ventricle

Ventral complex

Central Complex

10

Calcarine sulcus

Frontal lobe

4

Caudate

Internal ant. + ventral lat. complex

Posterior complex

Dorsal hippo-campus

6

Corona radiata

14

Globus pallidus

Interpeduncular nucleus

7

Basal ganglia

Occipital lobe

18

2 1

Anterior commissure

Cerebral peduncle

Ventral hippo-campus

3

Nucleus accumbens

Substantia innominata

Temporal lobe

Primary fissure

Ansiform lobule (crus I)

17

Orbital gyrus

12

Amygdala

11

9

Simplex lobule

Anterior lobe

Cerebellum (hemisphere)

Ansiform lobule (crus II)

13

10

Paramedian lobule

Primary olfactory cortex (piriform)

8 Parahippocampal gyrus

18

Biventral lobule

Lateral ventricle

Middle cerebellar peduncle

Paraflocculus?

Dentate nucleus?

Entorhinal cortex

Inferior cerebellar peduncle

Flocculus

PLATE 8A
CR 225 mm
GW 26, Y147-63
Sagittal
Section 321

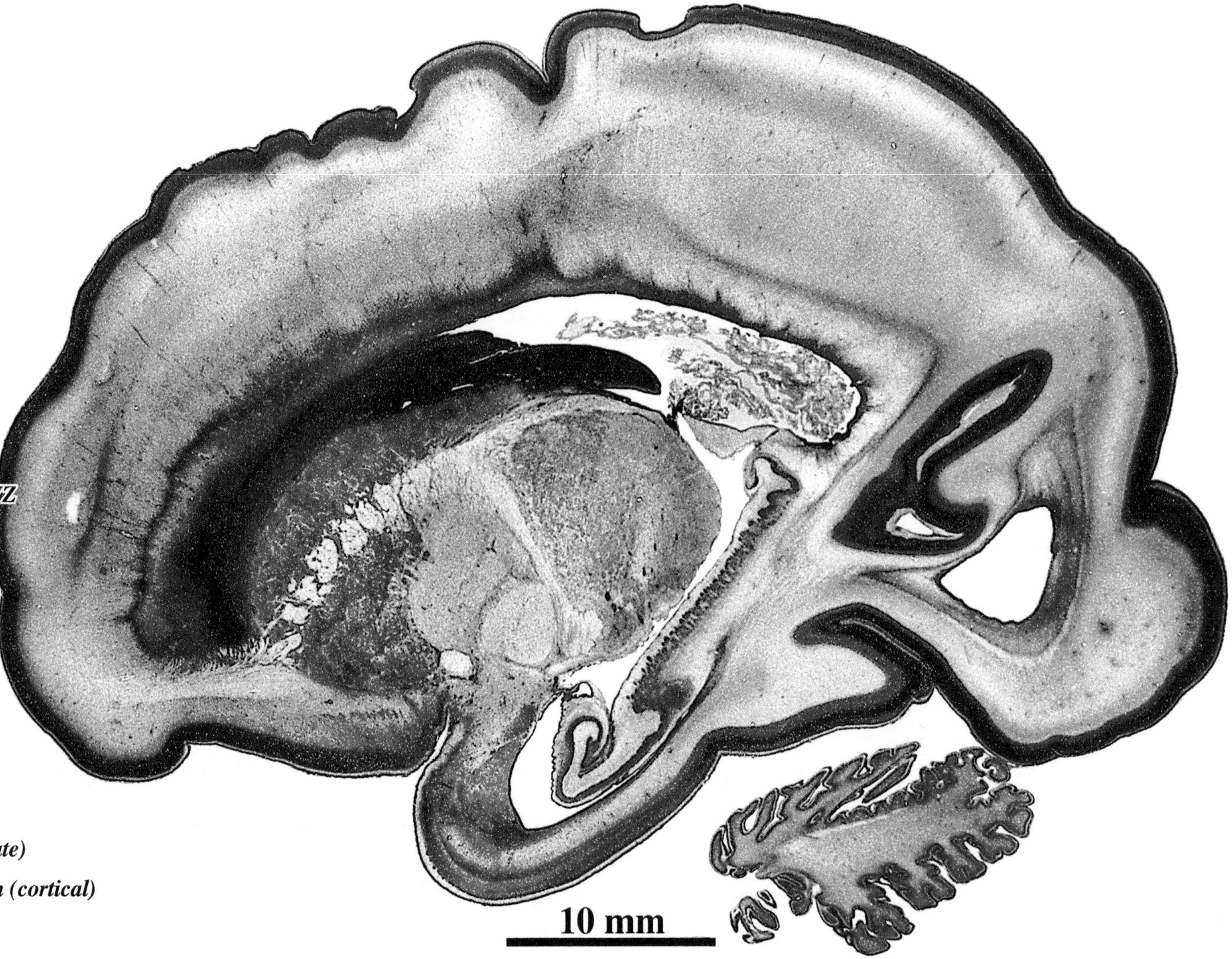

Remnants of the germinal matrix, migratory streams, and transitional fields

1 *Rostral migratory stream (source area)*
2 *Frontal NEP and SVZ*
3 *Frontal STF*
4 *Paracentral NEP and SVZ*
5 *Paracentral STF*
6 *Callosal GEP*
7 *Fornical GEP*
8 *Occipital NEP and SVZ*
9 *Occipital STF*
10 *Temporal NEP and SVZ*
11 *Temporal STF*
12 *Alvear GEP*
13 *Subgranular zone (dentate)*
14 *Lateral migratory stream (cortical)*
15 *Amygdaloid G/EP*
16 *Anterolateral striatal NEP and SVZ*
17 *Anteromedial/posterior striatal NEP and SVZ*
18 *Strionuclear GEP*
19 *External germinal layer (cerebellum)*
20 *Subpial granular layer (cortical)*

GEP - Glioepithelium
G/EP - Glioepithelium/ependyma
NEP - Neuroepithelium
STF - Stratified transitional field
SVZ - Subventricular zone

10 mm

See detail of the brain core and the cerebellum in Plates 18A and B.

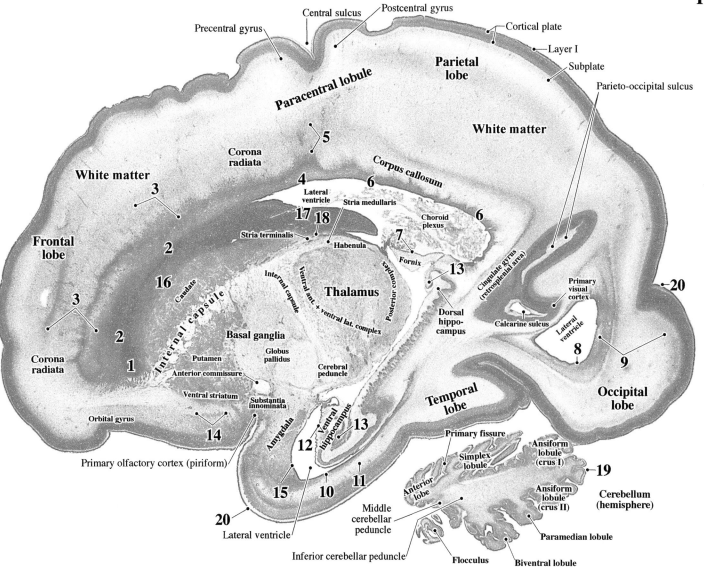

Precentral gyrus

Central sulcus

Postcentral gyrus

Cortical plate

Layer I

Parietal lobe

Subplate

Parieto-occipital sulcus

Paracentral lobule

White matter

5

Corona radiata

Corpus callosum

4

Lateral ventricle

6

White matter

White matter

3

Stria medullaris

6

Choroid plexus

17 **18**

Stria terminalis

2

Habenula

7

Fornix

Frontal lobe

16

Caudate

Internal capsule

Ventral ant. + ventral lat. complex

Thalamus

Posterior complex

13

Cingulate gyrus (retrosplenial area)

Primary visual cortex

20

3

Internal capsule

Basal ganglia

Dorsal hippo-campus

Calcarine sulcus

Lateral ventricle

2

Putamen

Globus pallidus

Cerebral peduncle

8

9

1

Corona radiata

Anterior commissure

Ventral striatum

Substantia innominata

Amygdala

Temporal lobe

Occipital lobe

Orbital gyrus

14

Ventral hippocampus

13

Primary fissure

Ansiform lobule (crus I)

Primary olfactory cortex (piriform)

12

10

11

Simplex lobule

19

15

Anterior lobe

Ansiform lobule (crus II)

Cerebellum (hemisphere)

20

Middle cerebellar peduncle

Paramedian lobule

Lateral ventricle

Inferior cerebellar peduncle

Flocculus

Biventral lobule

PLATE 9A
CR 225 mm
GW 26, Y147-63
Sagittal
Section 261

Remnants of the
germinal matrix,
migratory streams,
and transitional fields

1   *Frontal STF*

2   *Paracentral STF*

3   *Parietal NEP and SVZ*

4   *Parietal STF*

5   *Occipital NEP and SVZ*

6   *Occipital STF*

7   *Temporal NEP and SVZ*

8   *Temporal STF*

9   *Alvear GEP*

10 *Subgranular zone (dentate)*

11 *Lateral migratory stream (cortical)*

12 *Amygdaloid G/EP*

13 *Posterior striatal NEP and SVZ*

14 *Strionuclear GEP*

15 *External germinal layer (cerebellum)*

16 *Subpial granular layer (cortical)*

GEP - Glioepithelium
G/EP - Glioepithelium/ependyma
NEP - Neuroepithelium
STF - Stratified transitional field
SVZ - Subventricular zone

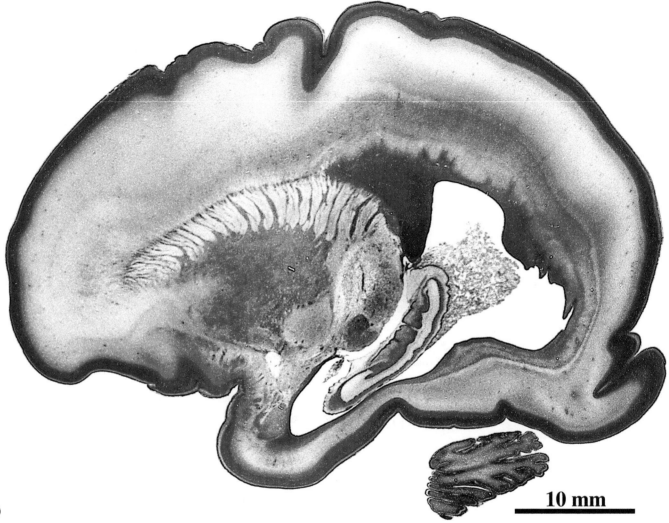

10 mm

See detail of the brain core in Plates 19A and B.

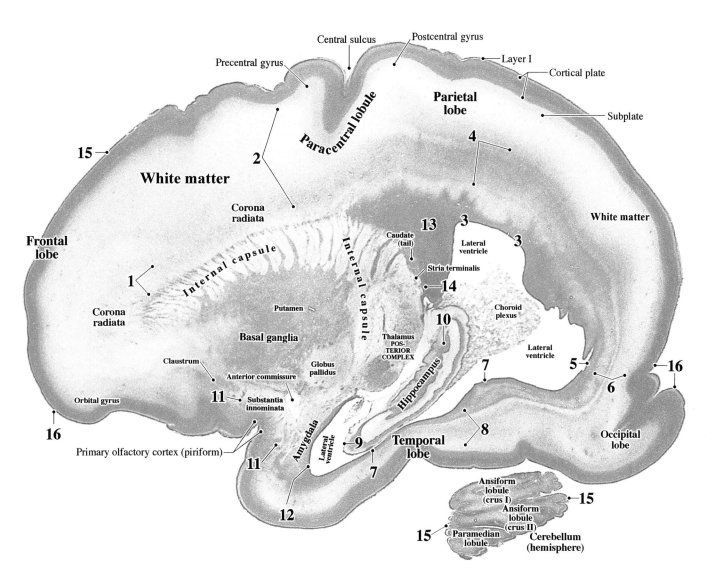

Central sulcus

Postcentral gyrus

Precentral gyrus

Layer I

Cortical plate

**Parietal
lobe**

Subplate

Paracentral lobule

15

2

4

White matter

Corona
radiata

13

3

Caudate
(tail)

Lateral
ventricle

3

White matter

**Frontal
lobe**

Internal capsule

Internal capsule

Stria terminalis

14

1

Putamen

Choroid
plexus

10

Corona
radiata

Basal ganglia

Thalamus
POS-
TERIOR
COMPLEX

Lateral
ventricle

Claustrum

Globus
pallidus

Hippocampus

7

5

16

Anterior commissure

11

Substantia
innominata

8

6

Orbital gyrus

Amygdala

Lateral
ventricle

9

**Temporal
lobe**

Occipital
lobe

16

Primary olfactory cortex (piriform)

11

7

Ansiform
lobule
(crus I)

15

12

Ansiform
lobule
(crus II)

15

Paramedian
lobule

Cerebellum
(hemisphere)

PLATE 10A
CR 225 mm
GW 26, Y147-63
Sagittal
Section 261

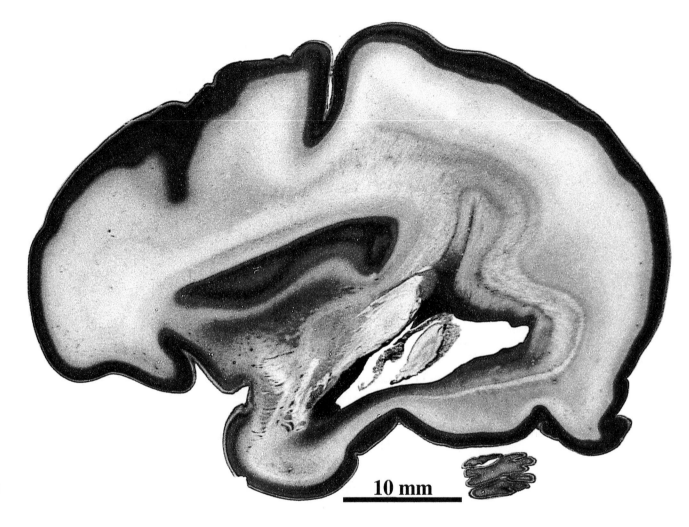

10 mm

Remnants of the
germinal matrix,
migratory streams,
and transitional fields

1 *Parietal NEP and SVZ*

2 *Parietal STF*

3 *Temporal NEP and SVZ*

4 *Temporal STF*

5 *Lateral migratory stream (cortical)*

6 *Amygdaloid G/EP*

7 *Posterior striatal NEP and SVZ*

8 *Strionuclear GEP*

9 *External germinal layer (cerebellum)*

10 *Subpial granular layer (cortical)*

GEP - Glioepithelium
G/EP - Glioepithelium/ependyma
NEP - Neuroepithelium
STF - Stratified transitional field
SVZ - Subventricular zone

See detail of the brain core in Plates 20A and B.

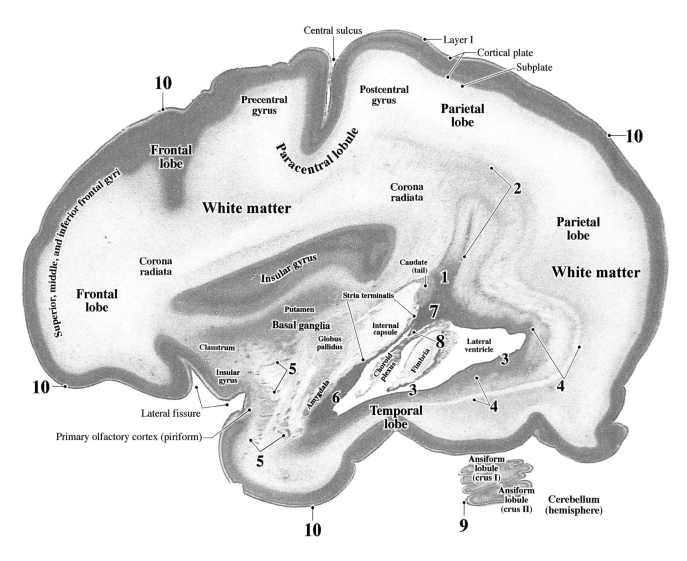

Central sulcus

Layer I

Cortical plate

Subplate

10

Precentral gyrus

Postcentral gyrus

Parietal lobe

10

Paracentral lobule

Frontal lobe

Superior, middle, and inferior frontal gyri

White matter

Corona radiata

2

Parietal lobe

Corona radiata

Insular gyrus

Caudate (tail)

White matter

Frontal lobe

Stria terminalis

1

Putamen

7

Basal ganglia

Internal capsule

Claustrum

Globus pallidus

8

Lateral ventricle

Insular gyrus

5

Choroid plexus

Fimbria

3

10

Amygdala

6

3

4

Lateral fissure

4

Temporal lobe

Primary olfactory cortex (piriform)

5

Ansiform lobule (crus I)

Ansiform lobule (crus II)

Cerebellum (hemisphere)

10

9

**PLATE 11A
CR 225 mm
GW 26, Y147-63
Sagittal
Section 501**

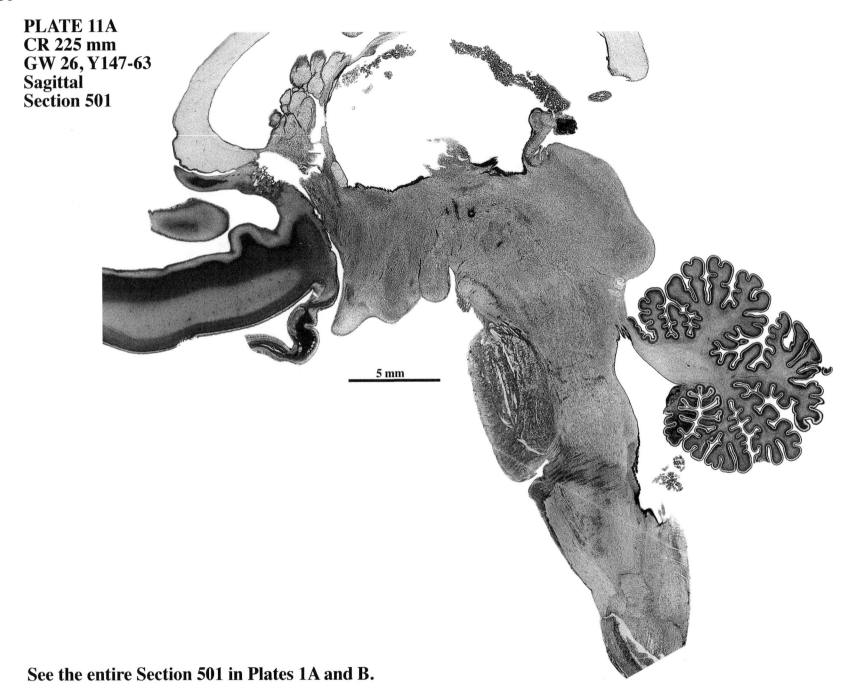

5 mm

See the entire Section 501 in Plates 1A and B.

31

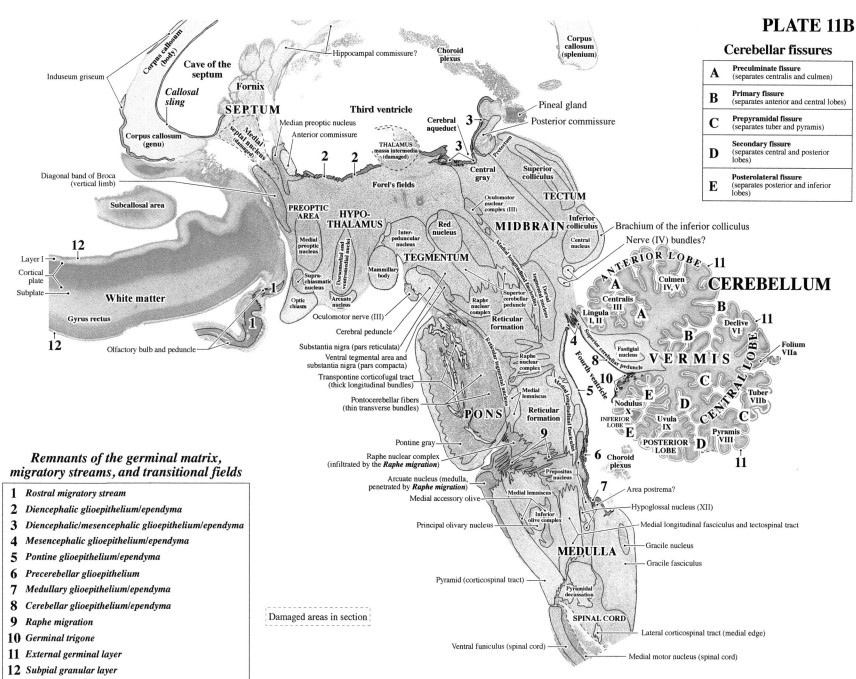

PLATE 11B

Cerebellar fissures

A	Preculminate fissure (separates centralis and culmen)
B	Primary fissure (separates anterior and central lobes)
C	Prepyramidal fissure (separates tuber and pyramis)
D	Secondary fissure (separates central and posterior lobes)
E	Posterolateral fissure (separates posterior and inferior lobes)

Remnants of the germinal matrix, migratory streams, and transitional fields

1 *Rostral migratory stream*
2 *Diencephalic glioepithelium/ependyma*
3 *Diencephalic/mesencephalic glioepithelium/ependyma*
4 *Mesencephalic glioepithelium/ependyma*
5 *Pontine glioepithelium/ependyma*
6 *Precerebellar glioepithelium*
7 *Medullary glioepithelium/ependyma*
8 *Cerebellar glioepithelium/ependyma*
9 *Raphe migration*
10 *Germinal trigone*
11 *External germinal layer*
12 *Subpial granular layer*

Damaged areas in section

PLATE 12A
CR 225 mm
GW 26, Y147-63
Sagittal
Section 481

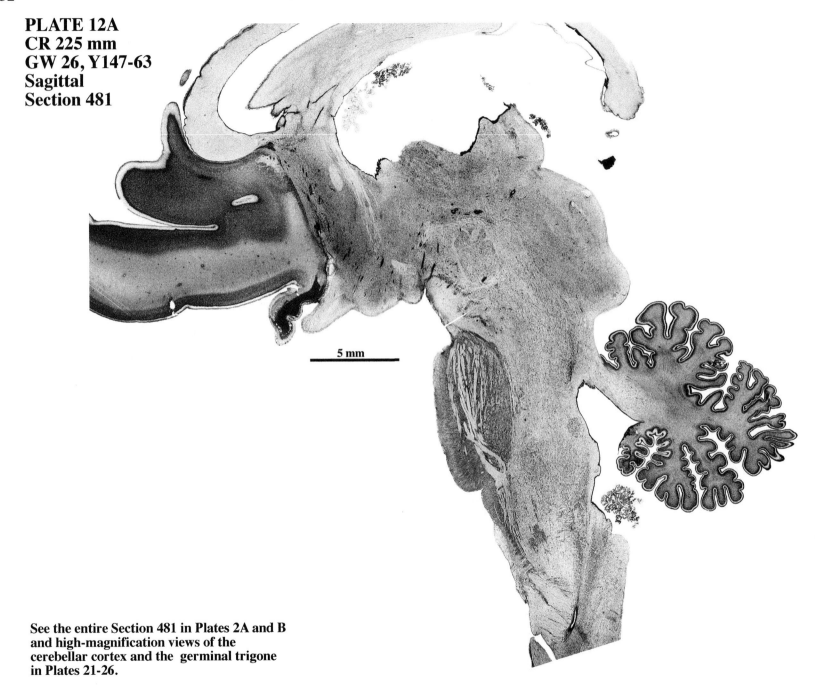

5 mm

See the entire Section 481 in Plates 2A and B
and high-magnification views of the
cerebellar cortex and the germinal trigone
in Plates 21-26.

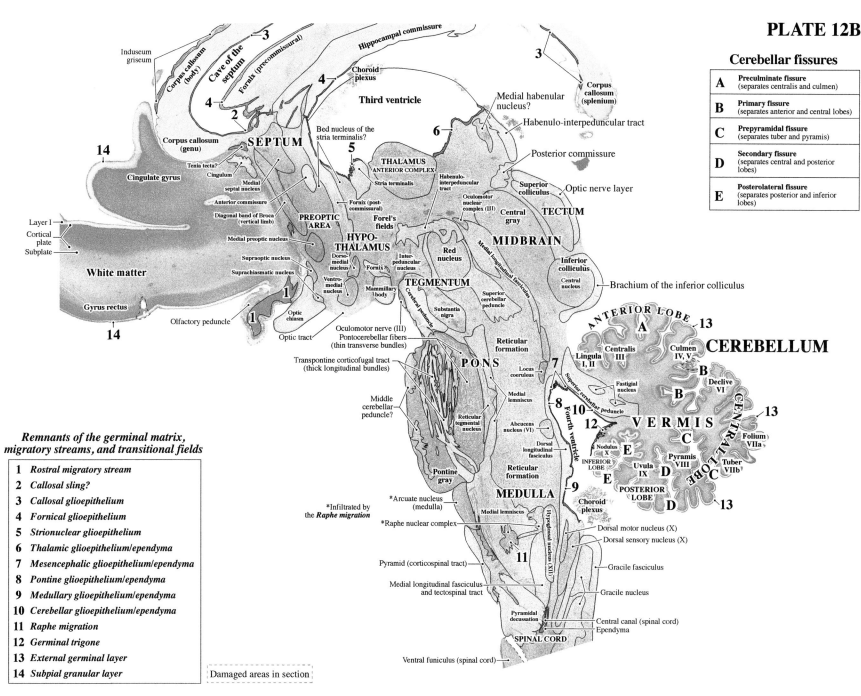

33

PLATE 12B

Cerebellar fissures

A	**Preculminate fissure** (separates centralis and culmen)
B	**Primary fissure** (separates anterior and central lobes)
C	**Prepyramidal fissure** (separates tuber and pyramis)
D	**Secondary fissure** (separates central and posterior lobes)
E	**Posterolateral fissure** (separates posterior and inferior lobes)

Remnants of the germinal matrix, migratory streams, and transitional fields

1 *Rostral migratory stream*
2 *Callosal sling?*
3 *Callosal glioepithelium*
4 *Fornical glioepithelium*
5 *Strionuclear glioepithelium*
6 *Thalamic glioepithelium/ependyma*
7 *Mesencephalic glioepithelium/ependyma*
8 *Pontine glioepithelium/ependyma*
9 *Medullary glioepithelium/ependyma*
10 *Cerebellar glioepithelium/ependyma*
11 *Raphe migration*
12 *Germinal trigone*
13 *External germinal layer*
14 *Subpial granular layer*

Damaged areas in section

PLATE 13A
CR 225 mm
GW 26
Y147-63
Sagittal
Section
461

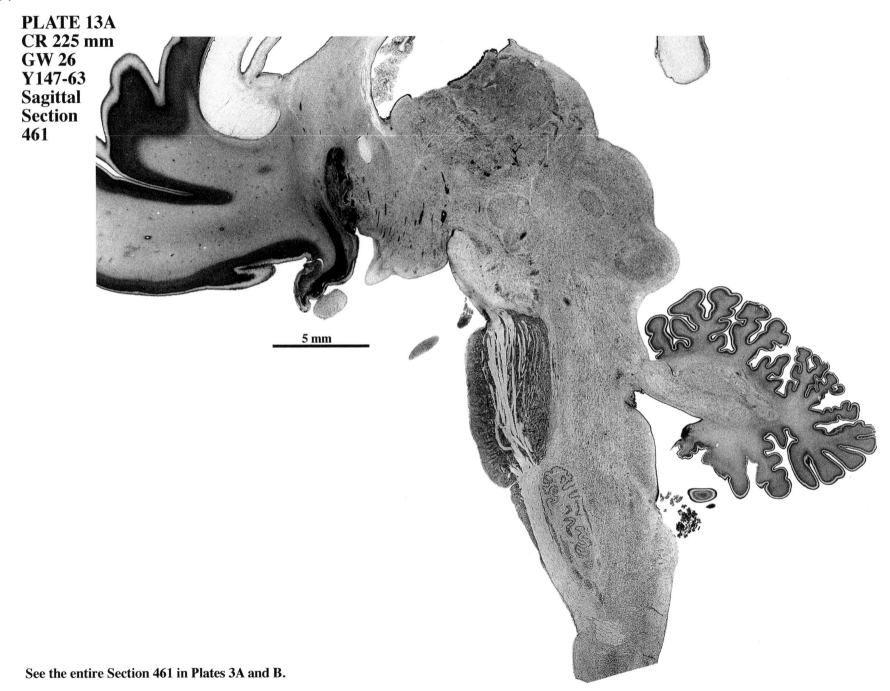

5 mm

See the entire Section 461 in Plates 3A and B.

PLATE 13B

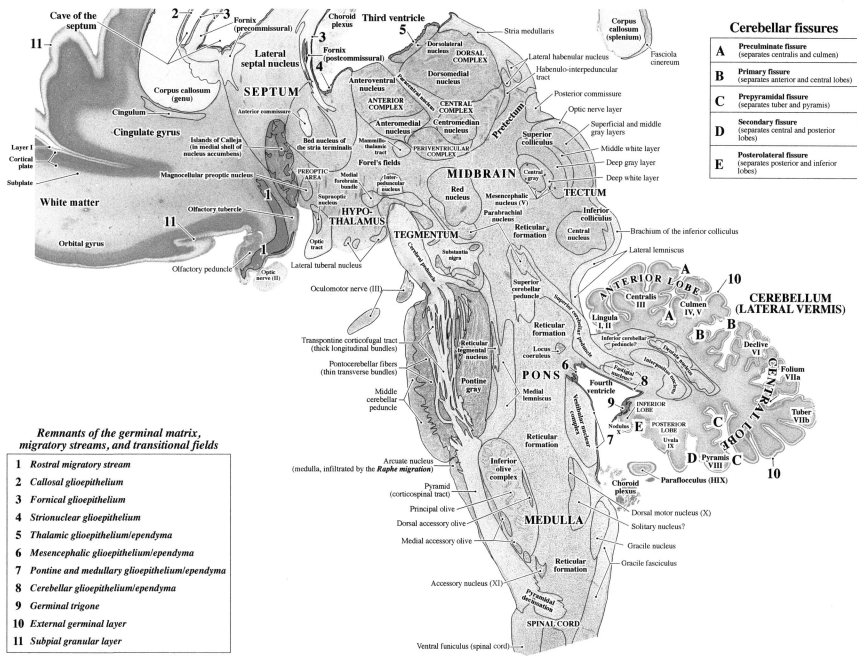

Cerebellar fissures

A	**Preculminate fissure** (separates centralis and culmen)	
B	**Primary fissure** (separates anterior and central lobes)	
C	**Prepyramidal fissure** (separates tuber and pyramis)	
D	**Secondary fissure** (separates central and posterior lobes)	
E	**Posterolateral fissure** (separates posterior and inferior lobes)	

Remnants of the germinal matrix,
migratory streams, and transitional fields

1 *Rostral migratory stream*

2 *Callosal glioepithelium*

3 *Fornical glioepithelium*

4 *Strionuclear glioepithelium*

5 *Thalamic glioepithelium/ependyma*

6 *Mesencephalic glioepithelium/ependyma*

7 *Pontine and medullary glioepithelium/ependyma*

8 *Cerebellar glioepithelium/ependyma*

9 *Germinal trigone*

10 *External germinal layer*

11 *Subpial granular layer*

Labels within figure:

Cave of the septum
11
Fornix (precommissural)
Choroid plexus
Third ventricle
5
Corpus callosum (splenium)
Stria medullaris
Fasciola cinereum
Dorsolateral nucleus
DORSAL COMPLEX
Lateral habenular nucleus
Habenulo-interpeduncular tract
Dorsomedial nucleus
Fornix (postcommissural)
Lateral septal nucleus
Anteroventral nucleus
Parcentral nucleus
CENTRAL COMPLEX
Posterior commissure
Corpus callosum (genu)
SEPTUM
ANTERIOR COMPLEX
Optic nerve layer
Cingulum
Anterior commissure
Anteromedial nucleus
Centromedian nucleus
Superficial and middle gray layers
Cingulate gyrus
Pretectum
Middle white layer
Layer I
Islands of Calleja (in medial shell of nucleus accumbens)
Bed nucleus of the stria terminalis
Mammillo-thalamic tract
PERIVENTRICULAR COMPLEX
Superior colliculus
Deep gray layer
Cortical plate
Forel's fields
Deep white layer
Subplate
Magnocellular preoptic nucleus
PREOPTIC AREA
Medial forebrain bundle
Inter-peduncular nucleus
MIDBRAIN
Central gray
White matter
Supraoptic nucleus
1
Red nucleus
TECTUM
Mesencephalic nucleus (V)
11
Olfactory tubercle
HYPO-THALAMUS
1
Optic tract
Parabrachial nucleus
Inferior colliculus
Orbital gyrus
TEGMENTUM
Substantia nigra
Reticular formation
Central nucleus
Brachium of the inferior colliculus
Olfactory peduncle
Lateral tuberal nucleus
Optic nerve (II)
Lateral lemniscus
Oculomotor nerve (III)
Cerebral peduncle
Superior cerebellar peduncle
ANTERIOR LOBE
A
10
Centralis III
A
Culmen IV, V
CEREBELLUM (LATERAL VERMIS)
Superior cerebellar peduncle
Lingula I, II
B
B
Transpontine corticofugal tract (thick longitudinal bundles)
Reticular tegmental nucleus
Reticular formation
Inferior cerebellar peduncle?
Dentate nucleus
Declive VI
Pontocerebellar fibers (thin transverse bundles)
Locus coeruleus
Interpositus nucleus
Folium VIIa
Pontine gray
6
Fastigial nucleus?
8
Middle cerebellar peduncle
Medial lemniscus
Fourth ventricle
9
INFERIOR LOBE
Vestibular nuclear complex
CENTRAL LOBE
PONS
Nodulus X
E
POSTERIOR LOBE
Tuber VIIb
Reticular formation
7
Uvula IX
Arcuate nucleus (medulla, infiltrated by the Raphe migration)
Inferior olive complex
Choroid plexus
D
Pyramis VIII
C
10
Pyramid (corticospinal tract)
Paraflocculus (HIX)
Principal olive
Dorsal motor nucleus (X)
Dorsal accessory olive
MEDULLA
Solitary nucleus?
Medial accessory olive
Gracile nucleus
Reticular formation
Gracile fasciculus
Accessory nucleus (XI)
Pyramidal decussation
SPINAL CORD
Ventral funiculus (spinal cord)

PLATE 14A
CR 225 mm
GW 26
Y147-63
Sagittal
Section
421

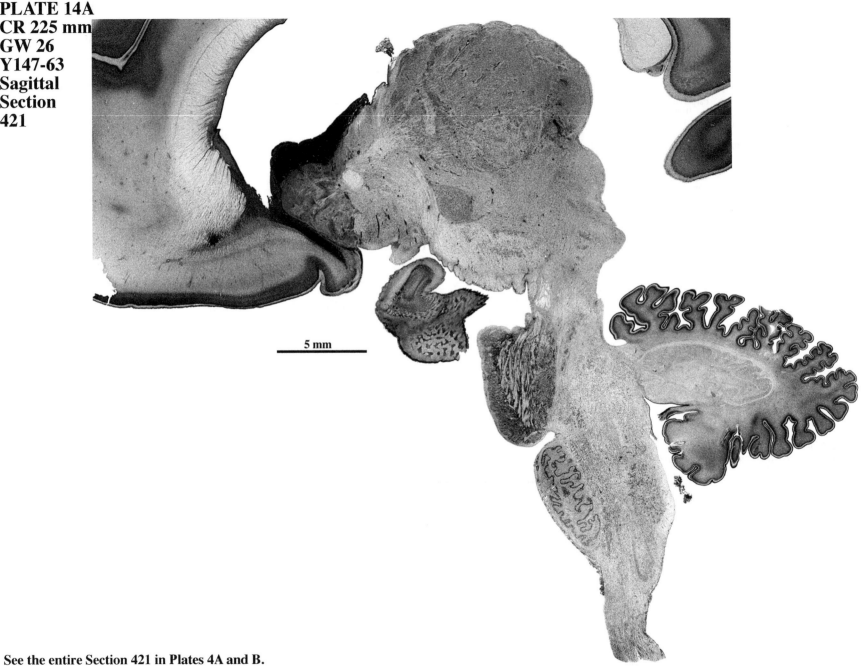

5 mm

See the entire Section 421 in Plates 4A and B.

37

PLATE 14B

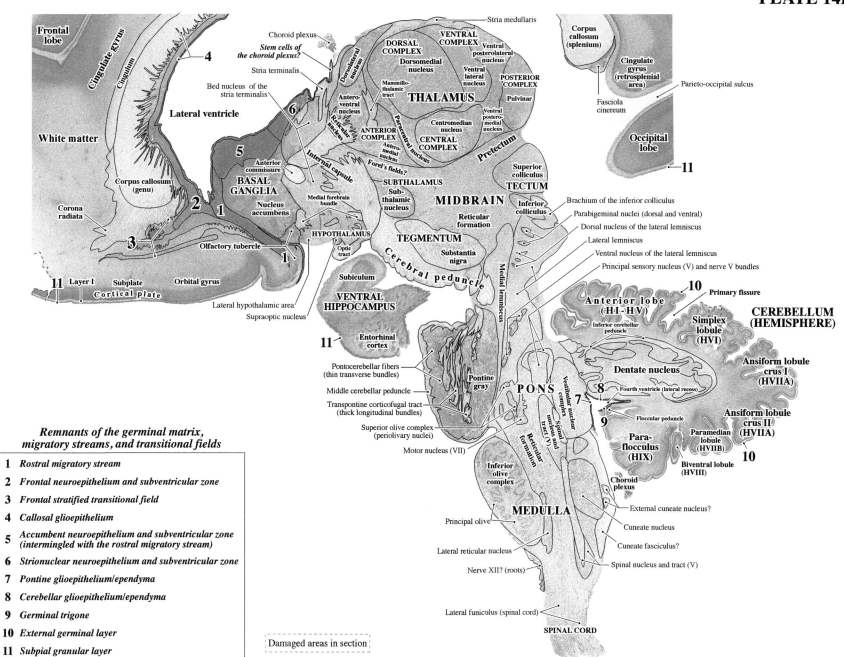

Remnants of the germinal matrix, migratory streams, and transitional fields

1 *Rostral migratory stream*
2 *Frontal neuroepithelium and subventricular zone*
3 *Frontal stratified transitional field*
4 *Callosal glioepithelium*
5 *Accumbent neuroepithelium and subventricular zone (intermingled with the rostral migratory stream)*
6 *Strionuclear neuroepithelium and subventricular zone*
7 *Pontine glioepithelium/ependyma*
8 *Cerebellar glioepithelium/ependyma*
9 *Germinal trigone*
10 *External germinal layer*
11 *Subpial granular layer*

Damaged areas in section

38

PLATE 15A, CR 225 mm, GW 26, Y147-63, Sagittal, Section 381

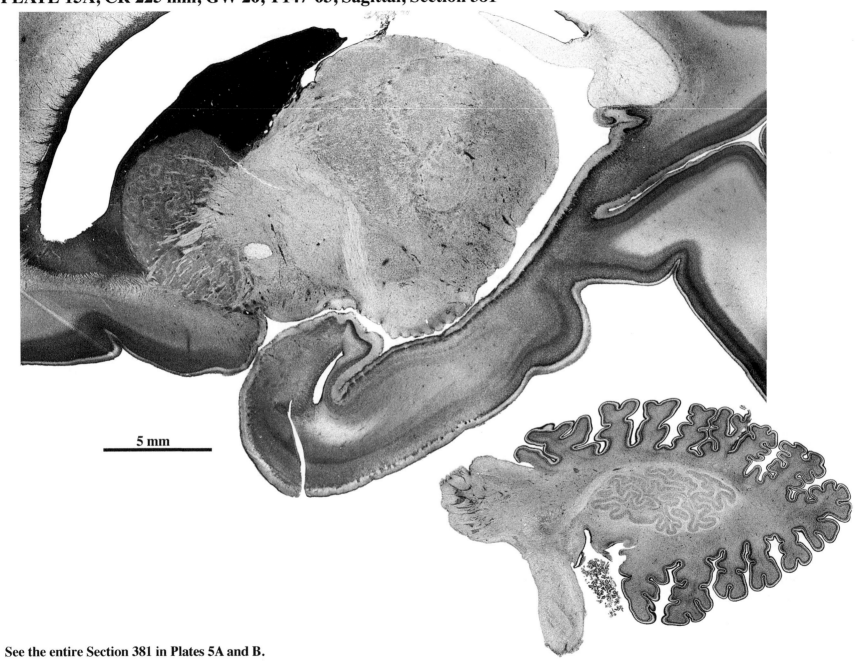

5 mm

See the entire Section 381 in Plates 5A and B.

Stem cells of the choroid plexus?

Choroid plexus

Fornix

Induseum griseum?

Corpus callosum

Lateral ventricle

DORSAL COMPLEX
Dorsolateral nucleus

VENTRAL COMPLEX

Corpus callosum (splenium)

Cingulum

Ventral postero-lateral nucleus

Ventral lateral nucleus

Central lateral nucleus

THALAMUS

Pulvinar

DORSAL HIPPO-CAMPUS

Cingulate gyrus (retrosplenial area)

Parieto-occipital sulcus

Cuneus

Stria terminalis

RETICULAR BELT

Ventral Anterior nucleus

CENTRAL COMPLEX

Centromedian nucleus

Lingula

Calcarine sulcus

Caudate (head)

Internal capsule (anterior limb)

Internal capsule
(Reticular nucleus)

BASAL GANGLIA

Paracentral nucleus

Ventral postero-medial nucleus

POSTERIOR COMPLEX

White matter

Occipital lobe

Globus pallidus (external segment)

Globus pallidus (internal segment)

SUBTHALAMUS

Medial geniculate body

Brachium of the inferior colliculus

Anterior commissure

Medullary lamina

Sub-thalamic nucleus

Zona incerta

Nucleus accumbens

Diagonal band of Broca (horizontal limb)

Substantia nigra

Olfactory tubercle

SUBSTANTIA INNOMINATA

Optic tract

Cerebral peduncle

Subplate

Cortical plate

Lateral olfactory tract

Corticomedial complex

Subiculum

Layer I

Primary olfactory cortex

Insular gyrus

VENTRAL HIPPOCAMPUS

Orbital gyrus

AMYGDALA

Basolateral complex

Parahippocampal gyrus

CEREBELLUM (HEMISPHERE)

Entorhinal cortex

Damaged area

Anterior lobe (HI-HV)

Primary fissure

Simplex lobule (HVI)

Ansiform lobule crus I (HVIIA)

Remnants of the germinal matrix, migratory streams, and transitional fields

Nerve V (root)

Dorsal cochlear nucleus

Dentate nucleus

1 *Rostral migratory stream (source area)*

2 *Frontal neuroepithelium and subventricular zone*

PONS

Middle cerebellar peduncle

Inferior cerebellar peduncle

Superior vestibular nucleus

Ansiform lobule crus II (HVIIA)

3 *Frontal stratified transitional field*

4 *Callosal glioepithelium*

5 *Fornical glioepithelium*

Ventral cochlear nucleus?

Fourth ventricle (lateral recess)

Floccular peduncle

6 *Parahippocampal neuroepithelium, subventricular zone, and stratified transitional field*

Para-flocculus (HIX)

Paramedian lobule (HVIIB)

7 *Alvear glioepithelium*

8 *Amygdaloid glioepithelium/ependyma*

Inferior cerebellar peduncle

Biventral lobule (HVIII)

9 *Anterolateral striatal neuroepithelium and subventricular zone*

10 *Anteromedial striatal neuroepithelium and subventricular zone*

Spinocerebellar tracts?

Choroid plexus

11 *Strionuclear glioepithelium*

12 *External germinal layer*

13 *Subpial granular layer*

Stem cells of the choroid plexus?

PLATE 16A
CR 225 mm
GW 26
Y147-63
Sagittal
Section 361

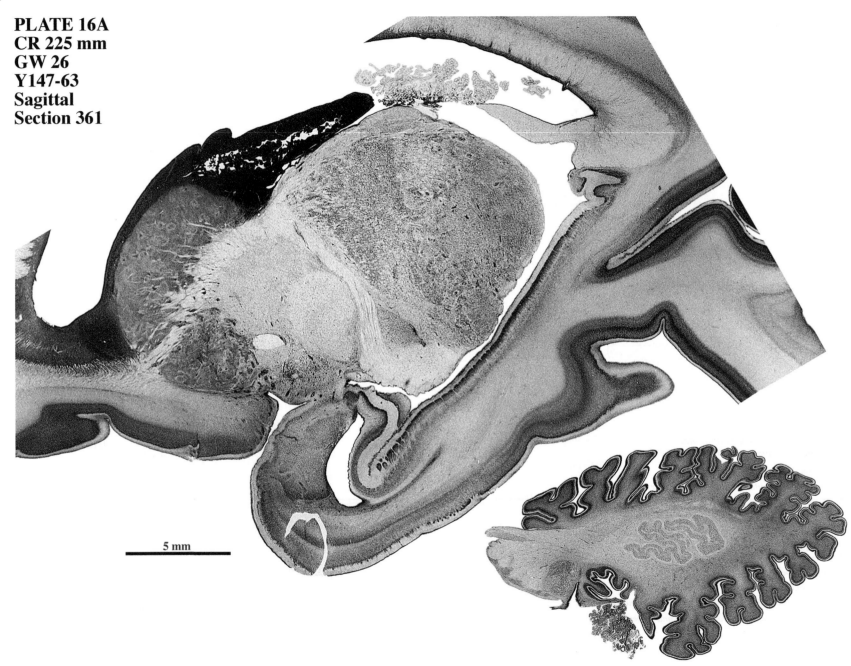

5 mm

See the entire Section 361 in Plates 6A and B.

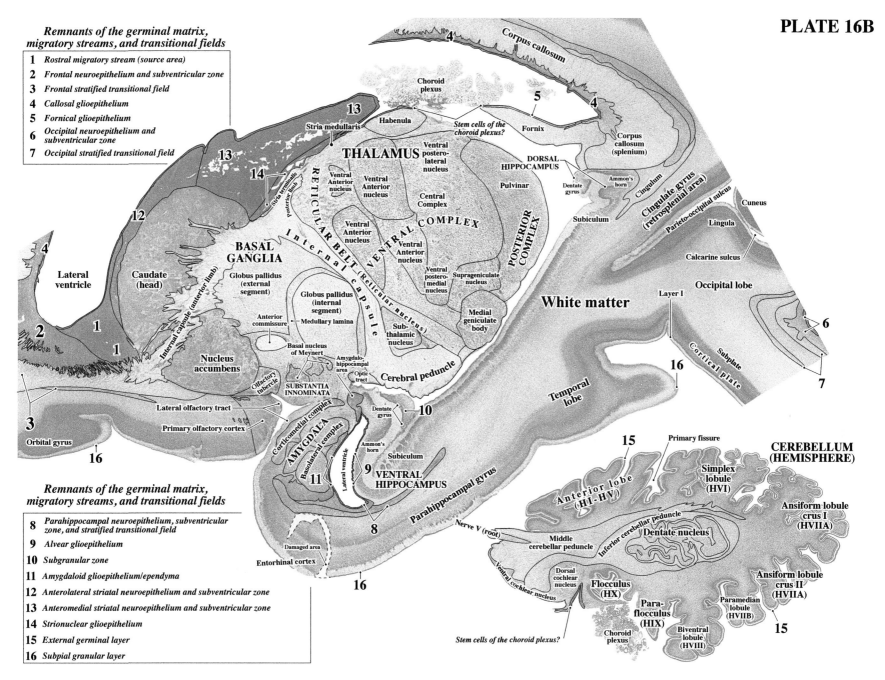

Remnants of the germinal matrix, migratory streams, and transitional fields

1 Rostral migratory stream (source area)
2 Frontal neuroepithelium and subventricular zone
3 Frontal stratified transitional field
4 Callosal glioepithelium
5 Fornical glioepithelium
6 Occipital neuroepithelium and subventricular zone
7 Occipital stratified transitional field

Remnants of the germinal matrix, migratory streams, and transitional fields

8 Parahippocampal neuroepithelium, subventricular zone, and stratified transitional field
9 Alvear glioepithelium
10 Subgranular zone
11 Amygdaloid glioepithelium/ependyma
12 Anterolateral striatal neuroepithelium and subventricular zone
13 Anteromedial striatal neuroepithelium and subventricular zone
14 Strionuclear glioepithelium
15 External germinal layer
16 Subpial granular layer

PLATE 17A
CR 225 mm
GW 26
Y147-63
Sagittal
Section 341

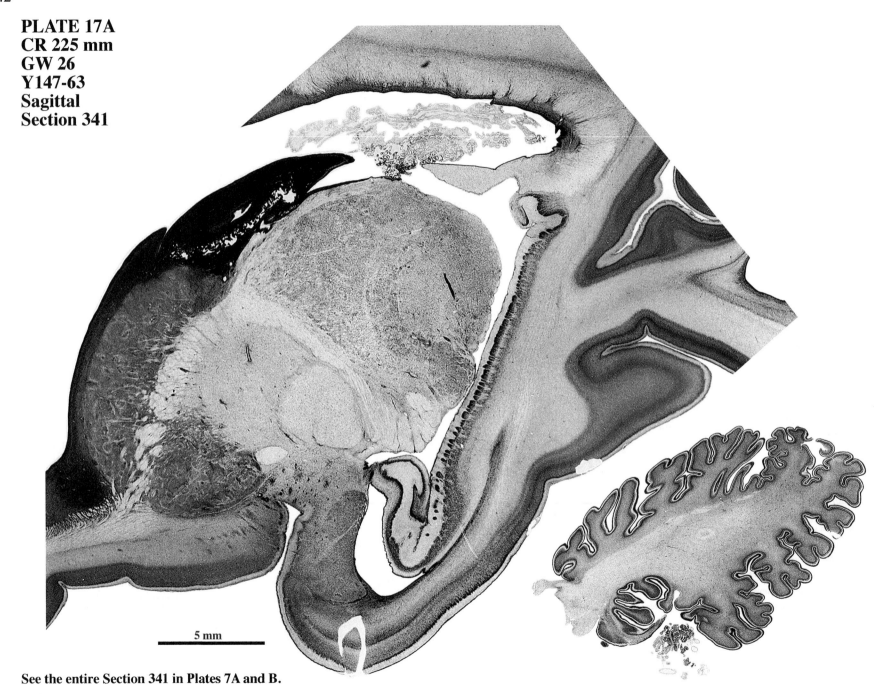

5 mm

See the entire Section 341 in Plates 7A and B.

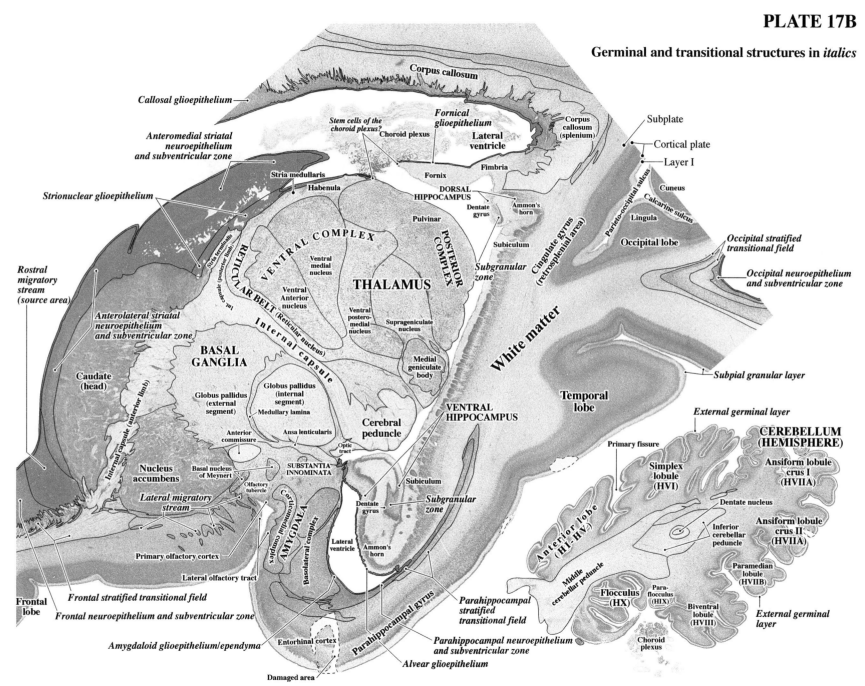

43

PLATE 17B

Germinal and transitional structures in *italics*

Callosal glioepithelium

Corpus callosum

Stem cells of the choroid plexus?

Choroid plexus

Fornical glioepithelium

Corpus callosum (splenium)

Subplate

Cortical plate

Layer I

Anteromedial striatal neuroepithelium and subventricular zone

Lateral ventricle

Fornix

Fimbria

DORSAL HIPPOCAMPUS

Stria medullaris

Habenula

Strionuclear glioepithelium

Dentate gyrus

Ammon's horn

Subiculum

Pulvinar

Cuneus

Calcarine sulcus

Lingula

Occipital lobe

Parieto-occipital sulcus

Occipital stratified transitional field

VENTRAL COMPLEX

Ventral medial nucleus

POSTERIOR COMPLEX

Subgranular zone

Cingulate gyrus (retrosplenial area)

Rostral migratory stream (source area)

RETICULAR BELT (Reticular nucleus)

Ventral Anterior nucleus

THALAMUS

Ventral postero-medial nucleus

Suprageniculate nucleus

Occipital neuroepithelium and subventricular zone

Anterolateral striatal neuroepithelium and subventricular zone

Int. capsule (posterior limb)

Internal capsule

Stria terminalis

Medial geniculate body

White matter

BASAL GANGLIA

Globus pallidus (external segment)

Globus pallidus (internal segment)

Medullary lamina

Cerebral peduncle

VENTRAL HIPPOCAMPUS

Temporal lobe

Subpial granular layer

Caudate (head)

Anterior commissure

Ansa lenticularis

SUBSTANTIA INNOMINATA

Optic tract

External germinal layer

Primary fissure

Simplex lobule (HVI)

CEREBELLUM (HEMISPHERE)

Ansiform lobule crus I (HVIIA)

Internal capsule (anterior limb)

Nucleus accumbens

Basal nucleus of Meynert

Olfactory tubercle

Subiculum

Subgranular zone

Dentate nucleus

Anterior lobe (HI–HV)

Ansiform lobule crus II (HVIIA)

Lateral migratory stream

Corticomedial complex

AMYGDALA

Basolateral complex

Dentate gyrus

Inferior cerebellar peduncle

Paramedian lobule (HVIIB)

Primary olfactory cortex

Lateral ventricle

Ammon's horn

Middle cerebellar peduncle

Flocculus (HX)

Para-flocculus (HIX)

Biventral lobule (HVIII)

External germinal layer

Lateral olfactory tract

Frontal stratified transitional field

Parahippocampal stratified transitional field

Frontal lobe

Frontal neuroepithelium and subventricular zone

Parahippocampal gyrus

Parahippocampal neuroepithelium and subventricular zone

Amygdaloid glioepithelium/ependyma

Entorhinal cortex

Choroid plexus

Alvear glioepithelium

Damaged area

PLATE 18A, CR 225 mm, GW 26, Y147-63, Sagittal, Section 341

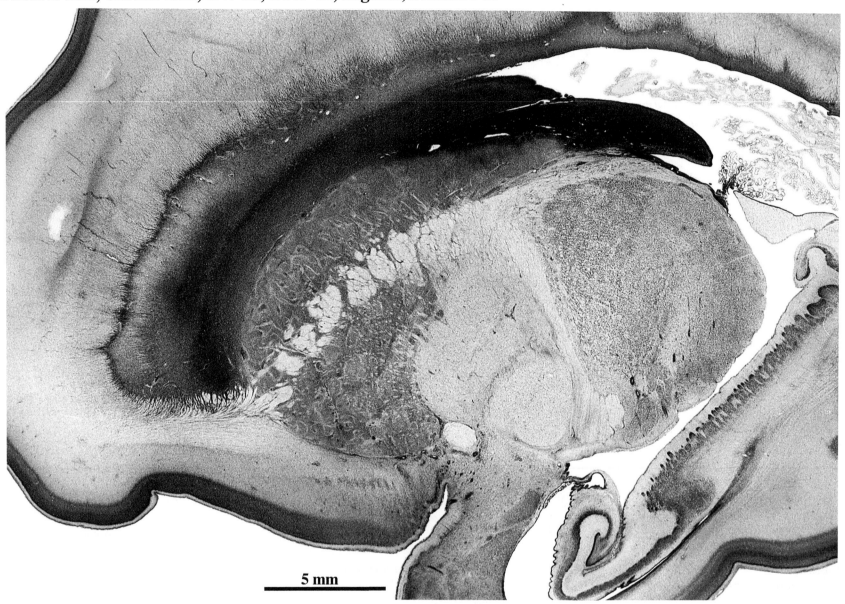

5 mm

See the entire Section 321 in Plates 8A and B.

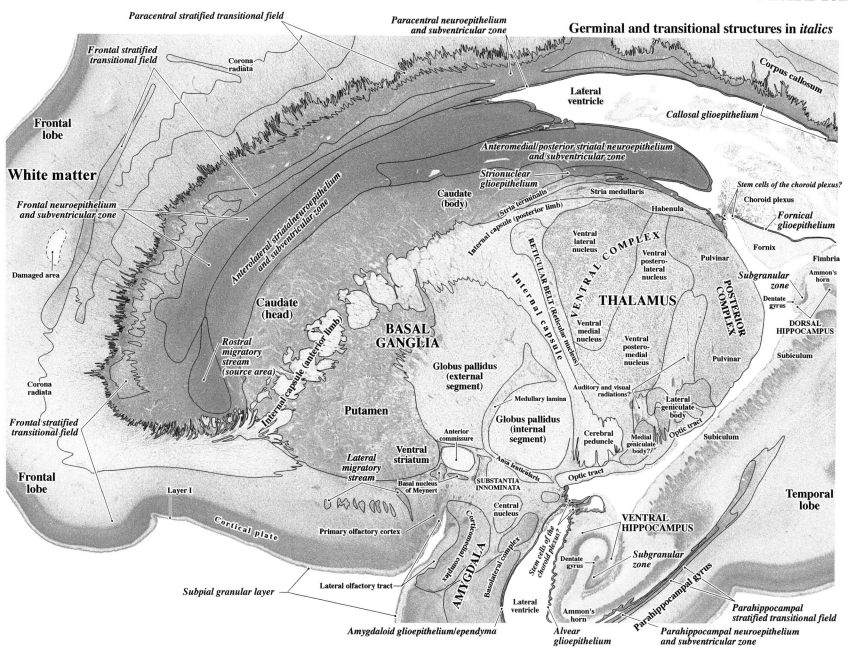

Germinal and transitional structures in *italics*

PLATE 19A
CR 225 mm, GW 26, Y147-63, Sagittal, Section 261

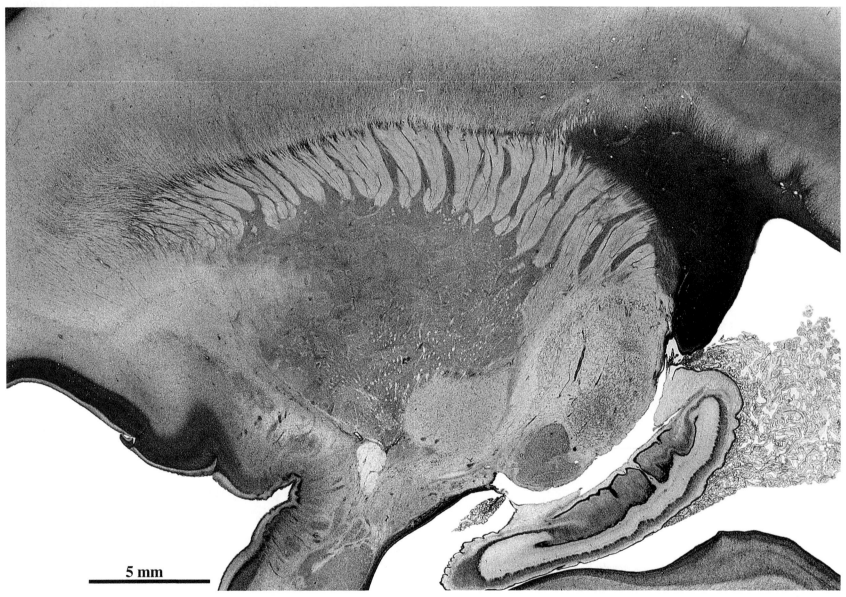

5 mm

See the entire Section 261 in Plates 9A and B.

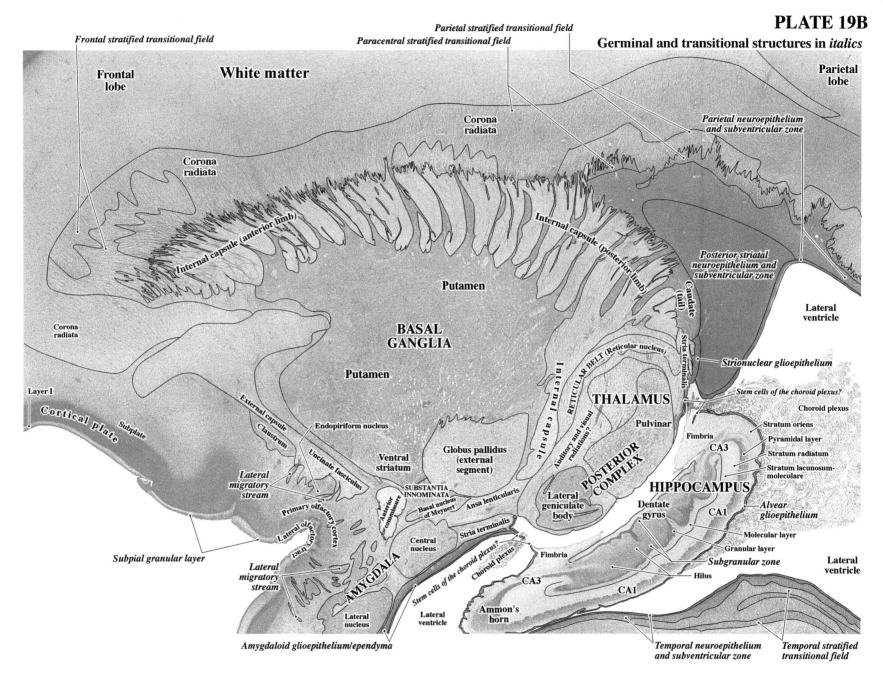

Germinal and transitional structures in *italics*

Frontal stratified transitional field

Parietal stratified transitional field
Paracentral stratified transitional field

Frontal lobe

White matter

Parietal lobe

Corona radiata

Corona radiata

Parietal neuroepithelium and subventricular zone

Internal capsule (anterior limb)

Corona radiata

Internal capsule (posterior limb)

Putamen

Posterior striatal neuroepithelium and subventricular zone

Caudate (tail)

Lateral ventricle

Corona radiata

BASAL GANGLIA

Putamen

RETICULAR BELT (Reticular nucleus)

Stria terminalis

Strionuclear glioepithelium

Layer I

External capsule

Endopiriform nucleus

THALAMUS

Stem cells of the choroid plexus?

Choroid plexus

Cortical plate

Subplate

Claustrum

Uncinate fasciculus

Ventral striatum

Globus pallidus (external segment)

Internal capsule

Auditory and visual radiations?

Pulvinar

Fimbria

CA3

Stratum oriens

Pyramidal layer

Stratum radiatum

Stratum lacunosum-moleculare

Lateral migratory stream

Primary olfactory cortex

SUBSTANTIA INNOMINATA

Basal nucleus of Meynert

Ansa lenticularis

POSTERIOR COMPLEX

Lateral geniculate body

HIPPOCAMPUS

Dentate gyrus

CA1

Alvear glioepithelium

Lateral olfactory tract

Subpial granular layer

Central nucleus

Stria terminalis

Molecular layer

Granular layer

Anterior commissure

Subgranular zone

Lateral ventricle

Lateral migratory stream

AMYGDALA

Lateral nucleus

Stem cells of the choroid plexus?

Choroid plexus

Fimbria

Hilus

CA3

CA1

Lateral ventricle

Ammon's horn

Lateral ventricle

Amygdaloid glioepithelium/ependyma

Temporal neuroepithelium and subventricular zone

Temporal stratified transitional field

PLATE 20A
CR 225 mm, GW 26, Y147-63, Sagittal, Section 221

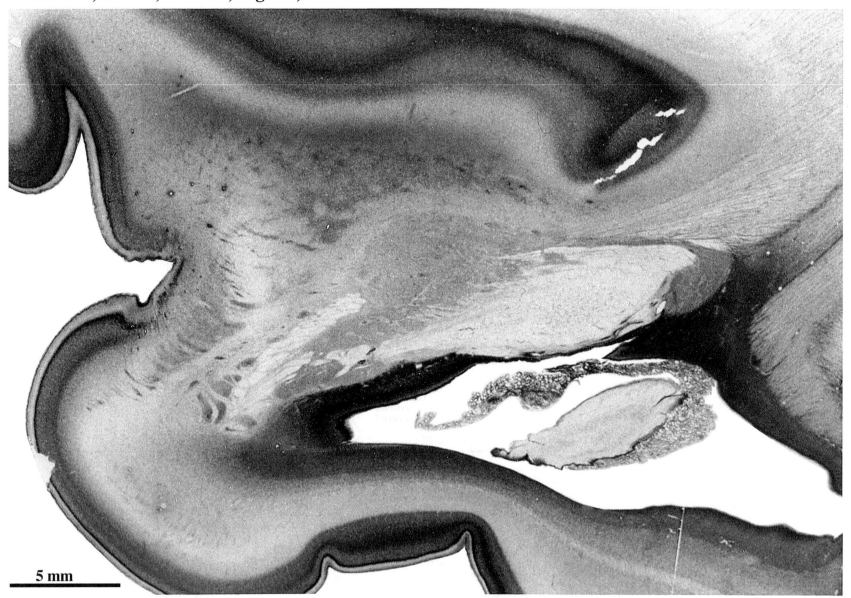

5 mm

See the entire Section 221 in Plates 10A and B.

Germinal and transitional structures in *italics*

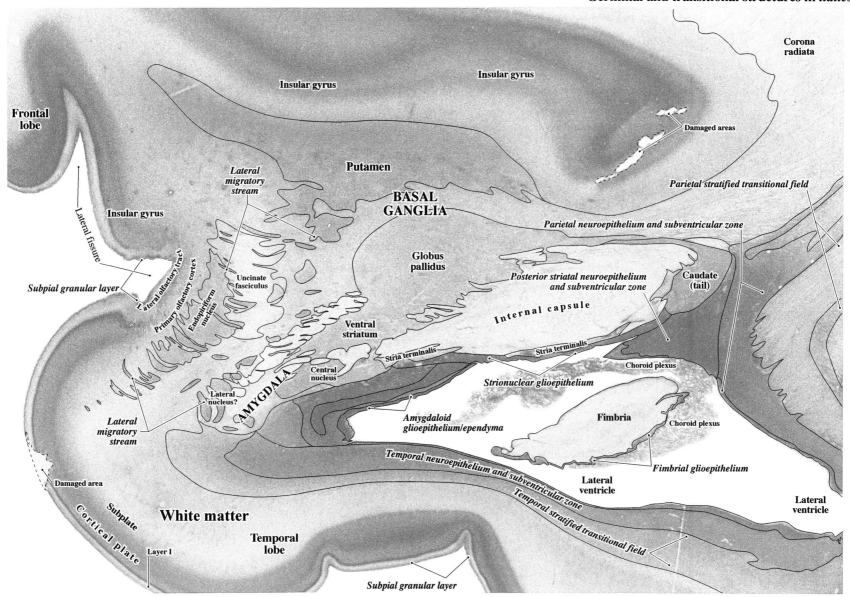

Corona radiata

Frontal lobe

Insular gyrus

Insular gyrus

Insular gyrus

Damaged areas

Parietal stratified transitional field

Lateral migratory stream

Putamen

BASAL GANGLIA

Parietal neuroepithelium and subventricular zone

Lateral olfactory tract

Primary olfactory cortex

Endopiriform nucleus

Uncinate fasciculus

Globus pallidus

Posterior striatal neuroepithelium and subventricular zone

Caudate (tail)

Lateral fissure

Subpial granular layer

Internal capsule

Ventral striatum

AMYGDALA

Central nucleus

Stria terminalis

Stria terminalis

Choroid plexus

Lateral nucleus?

Strionuclear glioepithelium

Lateral migratory stream

Amygdaloid glioepithelium/ependyma

Fimbria

Choroid plexus

Fimbrial glioepithelium

Temporal neuroepithelium and subventricular zone

Lateral ventricle

Damaged area

Lateral ventricle

Subplate

Cortical plate

White matter

Temporal stratified transitional field

Temporal lobe

Layer I

Subpial granular layer

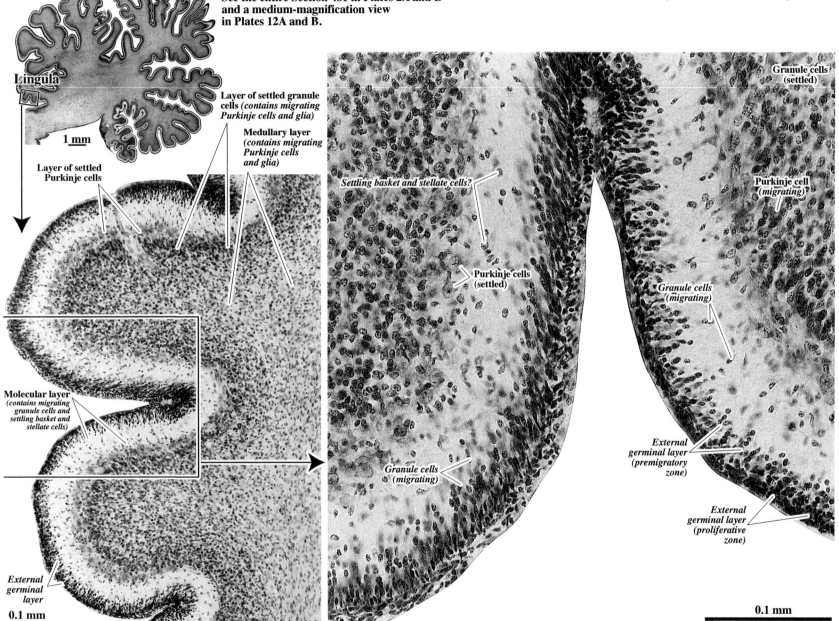

See the entire Section 481 in Plates 2A and B
and a medium-magnification view
in Plates 12A and B.

Lingula

1 mm

Layer of settled granule
cells (*contains migrating
Purkinje cells and glia*)

Medullary layer
(*contains migrating
Purkinje cells
and glia*)

Layer of settled
Purkinje cells

Molecular layer
(*contains migrating
granule cells and
settling basket and
stellate cells*)

*External
germinal
layer*

0.1 mm

Settling basket and stellate cells?

**Purkinje cells
(settled)**

*Granule cells
(migrating)*

Granule cells
(settled)

**Purkinje cell
(*migrating*)**

*Granule cells
(migrating)*

*External
germinal layer
(premigratory
zone)*

*External
germinal layer
(proliferative
zone)*

0.1 mm

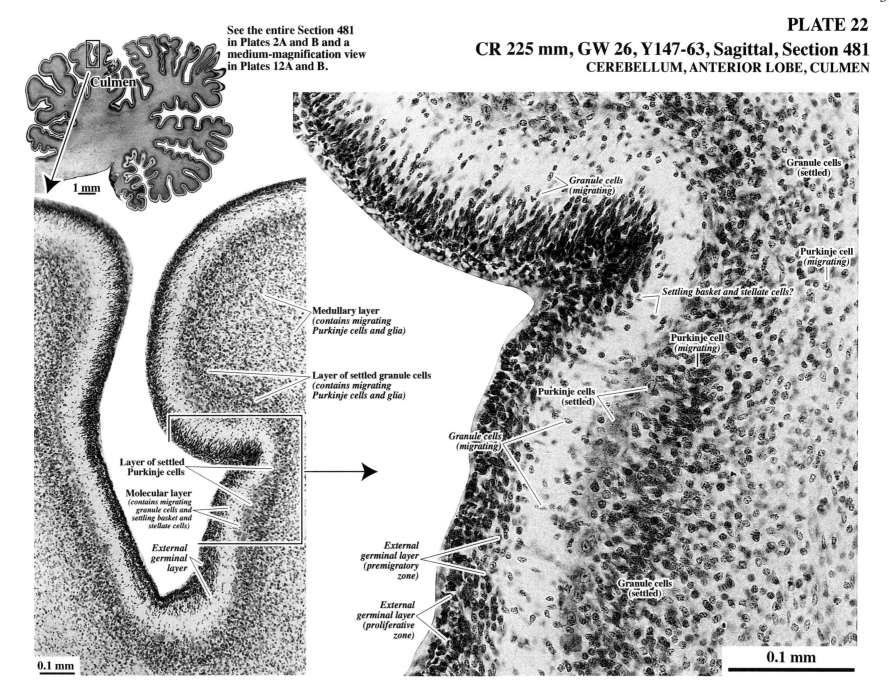

See the entire Section 481
in Plates 2A and B and a
medium-magnification view
in Plates 12A and B.

Culmen

1 mm

Granule cells
(migrating)

Granule cells
(settled)

Purkinje cell
(migrating)

Settling basket and stellate cells?

Purkinje cell
(migrating)

Medullary layer
(contains migrating
Purkinje cells and glia)

Purkinje cells
(settled)

Layer of settled granule cells
(contains migrating
Purkinje cells and glia)

Granule cells
(migrating)

Layer of settled
Purkinje cells

Molecular layer
(contains migrating
granule cells and
settling basket and
stellate cells)

External
germinal
layer

External
germinal layer
(premigratory
zone)

Granule cells
(settled)

External
germinal layer
(proliferative
zone)

0.1 mm

0.1 mm

52

PLATE 23

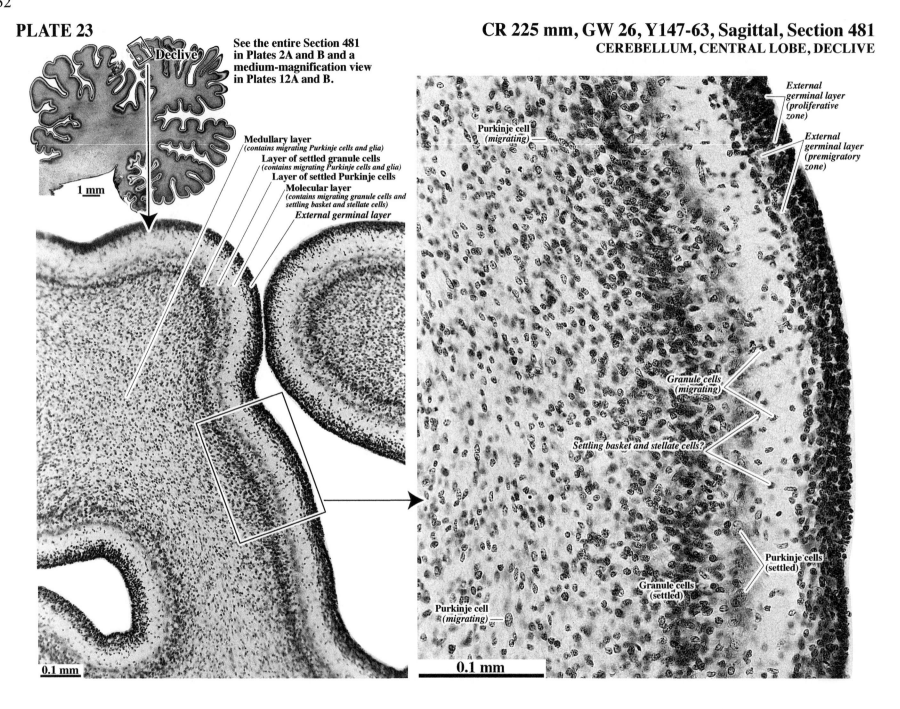

Declive

See the entire Section 481
in Plates 2A and B and a
medium-magnification view
in Plates 12A and B.

1 mm

Medullary layer
(contains migrating Purkinje cells and glia)
Layer of settled granule cells
(contains migrating Purkinje cells and glia)
Layer of settled Purkinje cells
Molecular layer
*(contains migrating granule cells and
settling basket and stellate cells)*
External germinal layer

0.1 mm

CR 225 mm, GW 26, Y147-63, Sagittal, Section 481
CEREBELLUM, CENTRAL LOBE, DECLIVE

*External
germinal layer
(proliferative
zone)*

*External
germinal layer
(premigratory
zone)*

Purkinje cell
(migrating)

*Granule cells
(migrating)*

Settling basket and stellate cells?

Purkinje cells
(settled)

Granule cells
(settled)

Purkinje cell
(migrating)

0.1 mm

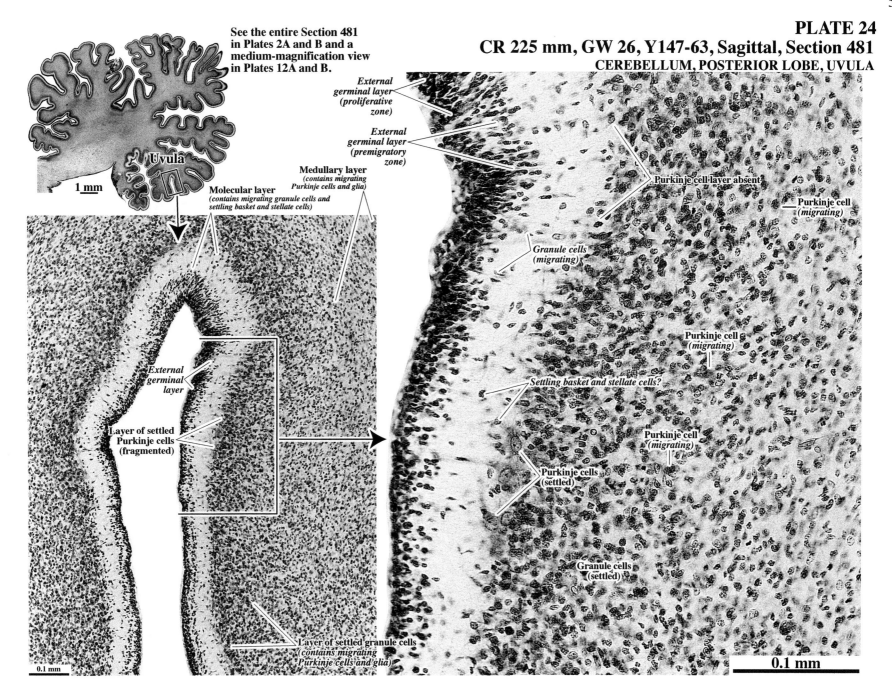

See the entire Section 481 in Plates 2A and B and a medium-magnification view in Plates 12A and B.

Uvula

1 mm

External germinal layer (proliferative zone)

External germinal layer (premigratory zone)

Purkinje cell layer absent

Purkinje cell (migrating)

Granule cells (migrating)

Purkinje cell (migrating)

Settling basket and stellate cells?

Purkinje cell (migrating)

Purkinje cells (settled)

Granule cells (settled)

Medullary layer (contains migrating Purkinje cells and glia)

Molecular layer (contains migrating granule cells and settling basket and stellate cells)

External germinal layer

Layer of settled Purkinje cells (fragmented)

Layer of settled granule cells (contains migrating Purkinje cells and glia)

0.1 mm

0.1 mm

54

PLATE 25

See the entire Section 481
in Plates 2A and B and a
medium-magnification view
in Plates 12A and B.

CR 225 mm, GW 26, Y147-63, Sagittal, Section 481
CEREBELLUM, INFERIOR LOBE, NODULUS

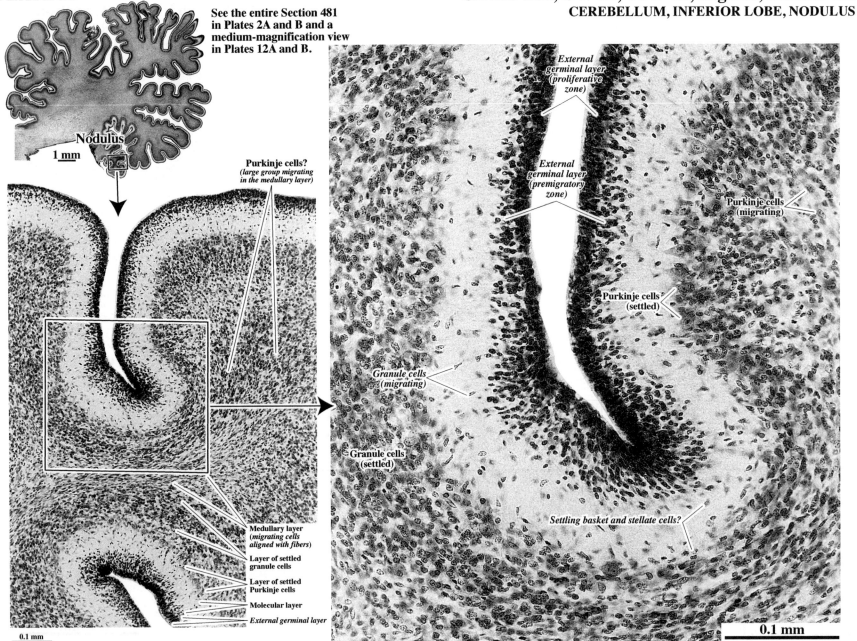

Nodulus

1 mm

Purkinje cells?
(large group migrating
in the medullary layer)

Medullary layer
(migrating cells
aligned with fibers)

Layer of settled
granule cells

Layer of settled
Purkinje cells

Molecular layer

External germinal layer

0.1 mm

External
germinal layer
(proliferative
zone)

External
germinal layer
(premigratory
zone)

Purkinje cells
(migrating)

Purkinje cells
(settled)

Granule cells
(migrating)

Granule cells
(settled)

Settling basket and stellate cells?

0.1 mm

PLATE 26

See the entire Section 481
in Plates 2A and B and a
medium-magnification view
in Plates 12A and B.

CR 225 mm, GW 26, Y147-63, Sagittal, Section 481
CEREBELLUM
Germinal Trigone

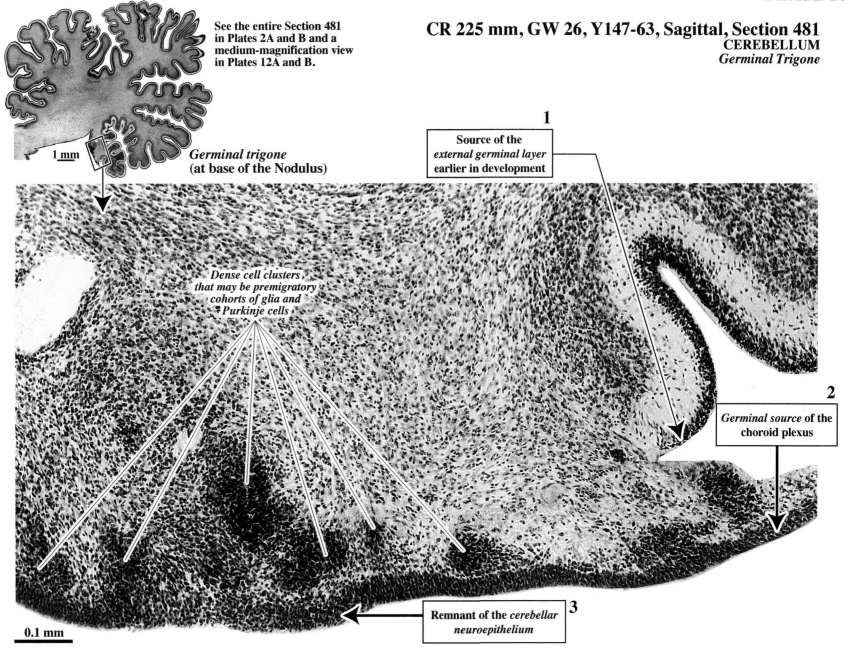

1 mm

Germinal trigone
(at base of the Nodulus)

1

Source of the
external germinal layer
earlier in development

*Dense cell clusters
that may be premigratory
cohorts of glia and
Purkinje cells*

2

Germinal source of the
choroid plexus

3

Remnant of the *cerebellar
neuroepithelium*

0.1 mm

PART III: Y16-59
CR 235 mm (GW 26)
Horizontal

This specimen is case number W-16-59 (Perinatal RPSL) in the Yakovlev Collection, a premature stillborn female infant. The brain is classified as a Normative Control in the Yakovlev Collection (Haleem, 1990). It was cut in the horizontal plane in 35-μm and 15-μm thick sections. Since there is no available photograph of this brain before it was embedded and cut, the photograph of the lateral view of another GW 26 brain that Larroche published in 1967 (**Figure 6**) is similar to the features of the brain in Y16-59.

The approximate cutting plane of this brain is indicated in **Figure 7** (facing page) with lines superimposed on the GW26 brain from the Larroche (1967) series. The anterior part of each section (on the left) is dorsal to the posterior part (on the right). As in all other specimens, the sections chosen for illustration are more closely spaced to show small structures in the diencephalon, midbrain, pons, and medulla. Illustrated sections are spaced farther apart when they contain only large brain structures, such as the cerebral cortex, basal ganglia, and cerebellum. Photographs of 15 Nissl-stained low-magnification sections are shown in **Plates 27-41**. **Plates 42-43** show the brainstem at high magnification because these sections are below the cerebral cortex. The core of the brain and the cerebellum are shown at high magnification in **Plates 44-56**.

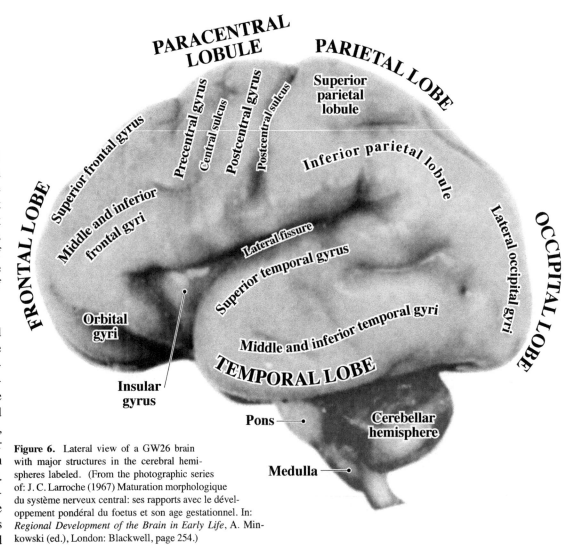

Figure 6. Lateral view of a GW26 brain with major structures in the cerebral hemispheres labeled. (From the photographic series of: J. C. Larroche (1967) Maturation morphologique du système nerveux central: ses rapports avec le développement pondéral du foetus et son age gestationnel. In: *Regional Development of the Brain in Early Life*, A. Minkowski (ed.), London: Blackwell, page 254.)

Y16-59 contains some prominent immature structures. A densely staining ***neuroepithelium/subventricular zone*** is generating neocortical interneurons and glia in all lobes of the cerebral cortex. Remnants of migrating and sojourning neurons and/or glia are also visible in all lobes of the cerebral cortex in ***stratified transitional fields***. Many neurons, glia, and their mitotic precursor cells are still migrating through the olfactory peduncle toward the olfactory bulb (***rostral migratory stream***) from a presumed source area in the germinal matrix at the junction between the cerebral cortex, striatum, and nucleus accumbens. Within the cerebral cortex, definite streams of neurons and glia are in the ***lateral migratory stream*** that percolates through the claustrum, endopiriform nucleus, external capsule, and uncinate fasciculus. These cells appear to be heading toward the insular cortex, primary olfactory cortex, temporal cortex, and basolateral parts of the amygdaloid complex. In the basal ganglia, there is a thick *neuroepithelium/subventricular zone* overlying the striatum and nucleus accumbens where neurons are being generated; at least three subdivisions (anteromedial, anterolateral, and posterior) can be distinguished in the striatum. Another region of active neurogenesis in the telencephalon is the *subgranular zone* in the hilus of the dentate gyrus that is the source of granule cells. Other structures in the telencephalon, such as the septum, fornix, and Ammon's horn part of the hippocampus, have only a thin, darkly staining layer at the ventricle, and these are presumed to be generating glia, cells of the choroid plexus, and the ependymal lining of the ventricle.

Most of the structures in the diencephalon appear to be settled and are maturing. The third ventricle is lined by a *glioepithelium/ependyma*. A convoluted *glioepithelium/ependyma* lines the cerebral aqueduct in the midbrain that continues into the anterior fourth ventricle. A smooth *glioepithelium/ependyma* lines the posterior fourth ventricle through the remainder of the pons and medulla. A convoluted *glioepithelium/ependyma* lines the floor of the fourth ventricle throughout the medulla.In the lower medulla and spinal cord, this specimen is remarkable for showing dense myelination gliosis in the cuneate fasciculus.

The *external germinal layer* covering the cerebellar cortex is actively producing basket, stellate, and granule cells. It is one prong of the *germinal trigone* at the base of the nodulus and along the floccular peduncle. Another prong is choroid plexus stem cells. The third prong is the *glioepithelium/ependym* beneath the cerebellum.

GW 26 HORIZONTAL SECTION PLANES

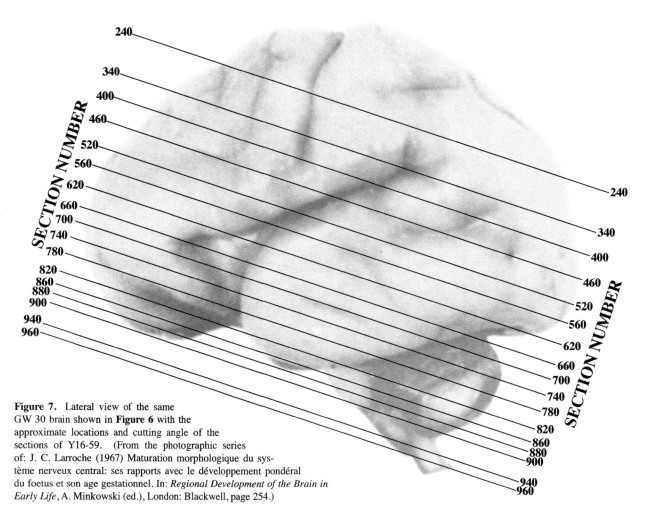

Figure 7. Lateral view of the same GW 30 brain shown in **Figure 6** with the approximate locations and cutting angle of the sections of Y16-59. (From the photographic series of: J. C. Larroche (1967) Maturation morphologique du système nerveux central: ses rapports avec le développement pondéral du foetus et son age gestationnel. In: *Regional Development of the Brain in Early Life*, A. Minkowski (ed.), London: Blackwell, page 254.)

PLATE 27A
CR 235 mm
GW 26, Y16-59
Horizontal
Section 240

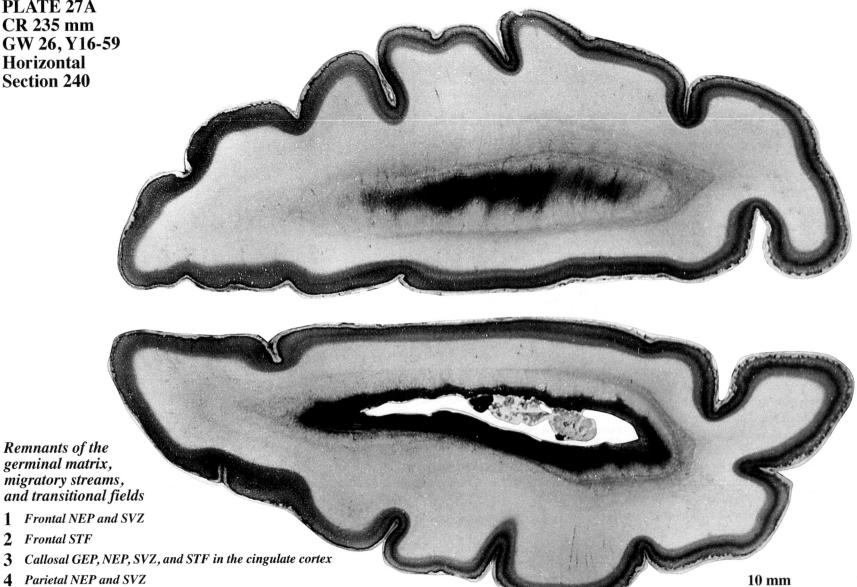

Remnants of the
germinal matrix,
migratory streams,
and transitional fields

1 *Frontal NEP and SVZ*

2 *Frontal STF*

3 *Callosal GEP, NEP, SVZ, and STF in the cingulate cortex*

4 *Parietal NEP and SVZ*

5 *Parietal STF*

6 *Paracentral NEP and SVZ*

7 *Paracentral STF*

8 *Subpial granular layer (cortical)*

GEP - Glioepithelium

NEP - Neuroepithelium

STF - Stratified transitional field

SVZ - Subventricular zone

10 mm

59

PLATE 27B

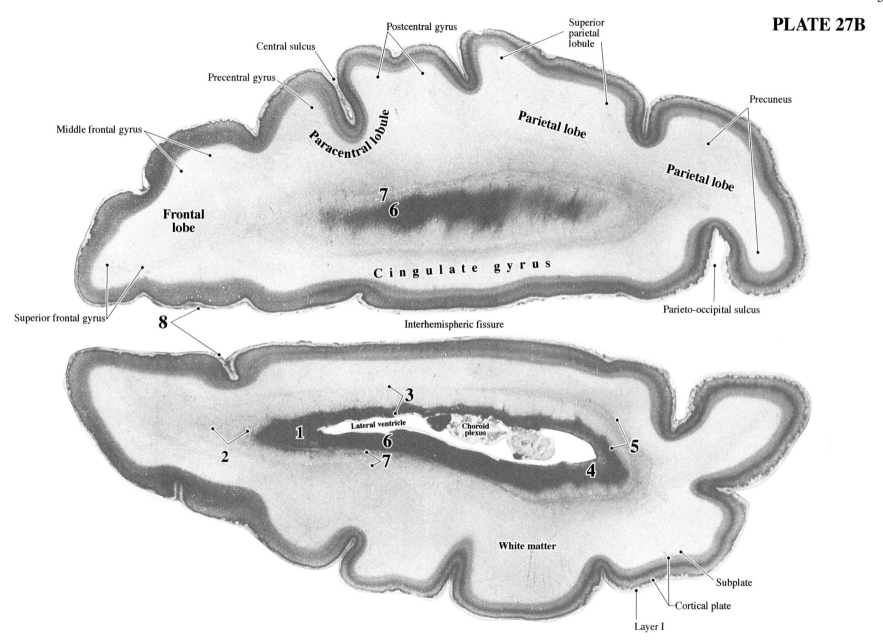

60

PLATE 28A
CR 235 mm
GW 26, Y16-59
Horizontal
Section 340

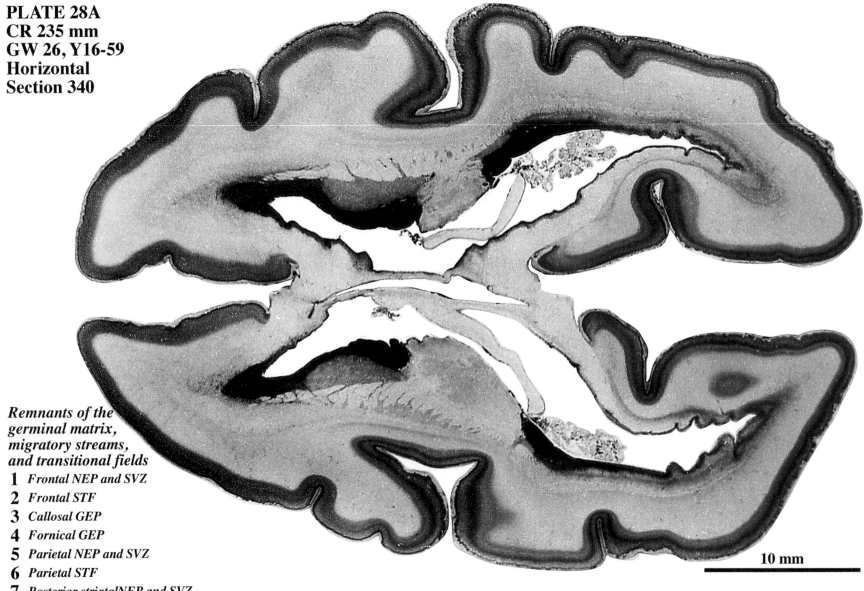

Remnants of the
germinal matrix,
migratory streams,
and transitional fields

1 *Frontal NEP and SVZ*
2 *Frontal STF*
3 *Callosal GEP*
4 *Fornical GEP*
5 *Parietal NEP and SVZ*
6 *Parietal STF*
7 *Posterior striatalNEP and SVZ*
8 *Anterolateral striatal NEP and SVZ*
9 *Anteromedial striatal NEP and SVZ*
10 *Strionuclear GEP*
11 *Subpial granular layer (cortical)*

GEP - Glioepithelium
NEP - Neuroepithelium
STF - Stratified transitional field
SVZ - Subventricular zone

10 mm

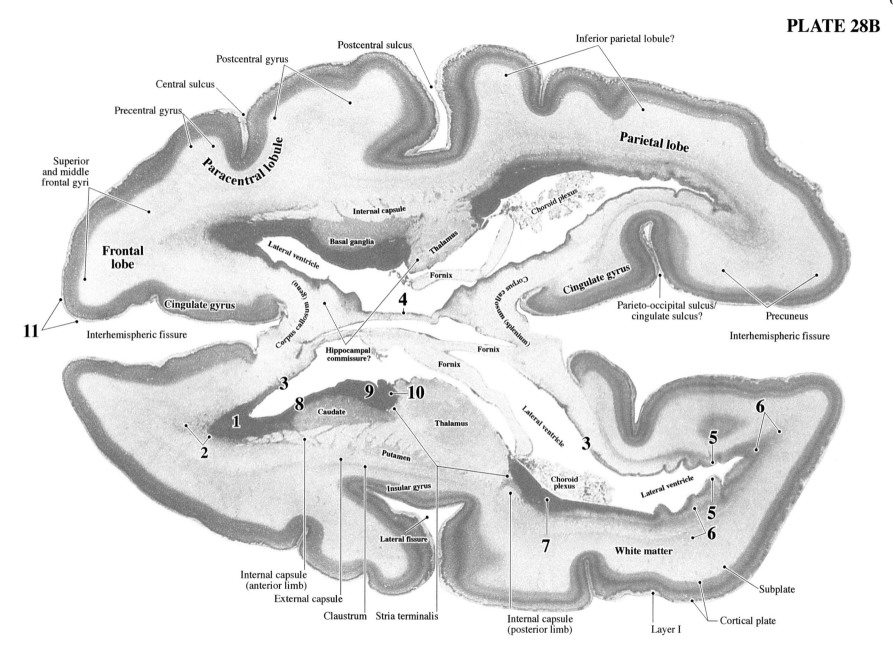

Postcentral sulcus

Inferior parietal lobule?

Postcentral gyrus

Central sulcus

Precentral gyrus

Parietal lobe

Superior
and middle
frontal gyri

Paracentral lobule

Internal capsule

Choroid plexus

Basal ganglia

Thalamus

Lateral ventricle

**Frontal
lobe**

Corpus callosum (genu)

Fornix

Corpus callosum (splenium)

Cingulate gyrus

Cingulate gyrus

4

Parieto-occipital sulcus/
cingulate sulcus?

11

Hippocampal
commissure?

Fornix

Precuneus

Interhemispheric fissure

Fornix

Interhemispheric fissure

3

9   **10**

6

8

Caudate

Lateral ventricle

1

Thalamus

3

5

2

Putamen

Insular gyrus

Choroid
plexus

Lateral ventricle

5

Lateral fissure

6

7

White matter

Internal capsule
(anterior limb)

Subplate

External capsule

Claustrum   Stria terminalis

Internal capsule
(posterior limb)

Layer I

Cortical plate

62

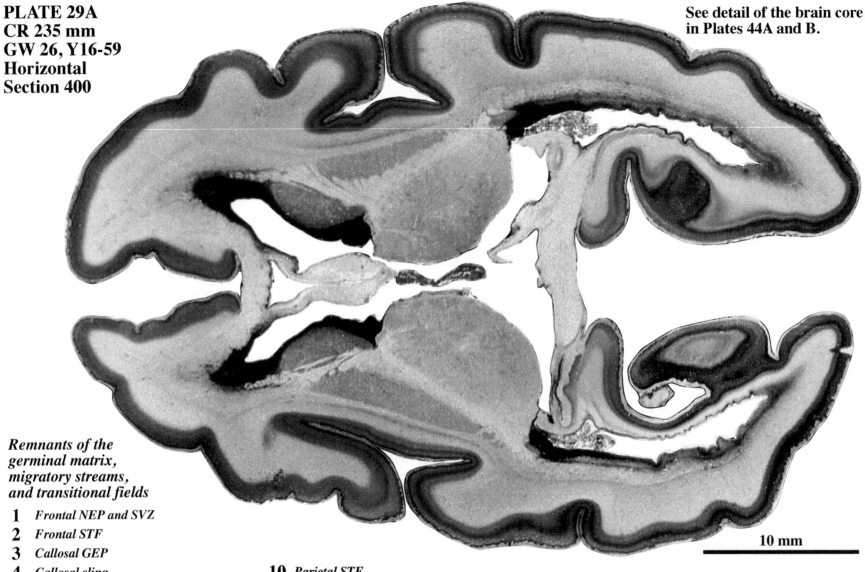

PLATE 29A
CR 235 mm
GW 26, Y16-59
Horizontal
Section 400

See detail of the brain core
in Plates 44A and B.

10 mm

Remnants of the
germinal matrix,
migratory streams,
and transitional fields

1   *Frontal NEP and SVZ*
2   *Frontal STF*
3   *Callosal GEP*
4   *Callosal sling*
5   *Fornical GEP*
6   *Parahippocampal NEP, SVZ, and STF*
7   *Occipital NEP and SVZ*
8   *Occipital STF*
9   *Parietal NEP and SVZ*

10 *Parietal STF*
11 *Posterior striatal NEP and SVZ*
12 *Anterolateral striatal NEP and SVZ*
13 *Anteromedial striatal NEP and SVZ*
14 *Strionuclear GE*
15 *Subpial granular layer (cortical)*

GEP - Glioepithelium
NEP - Neuroepithelium
STF - Stratified transitional field
SVZ - Subventricular zone

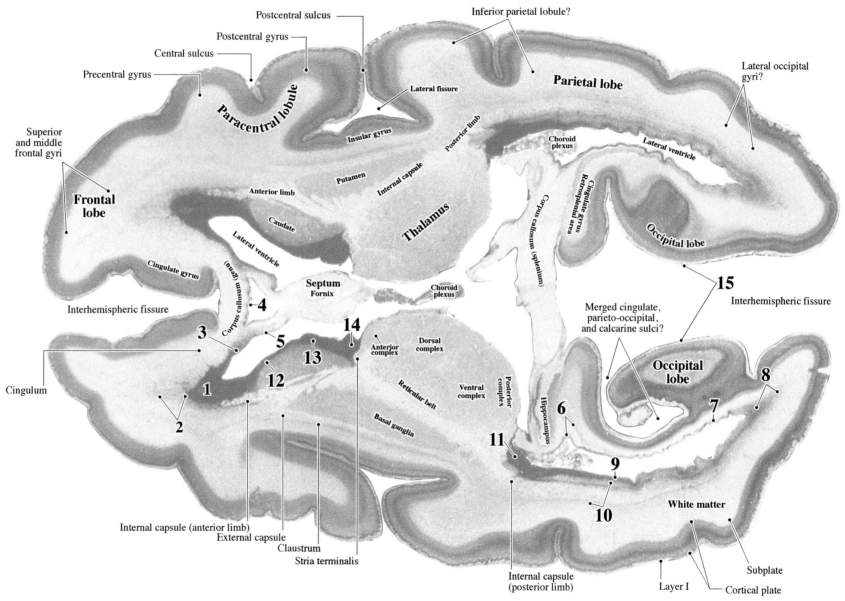

Postcentral sulcus

Postcentral gyrus

Central sulcus

Inferior parietal lobule?

Precentral gyrus

Lateral occipital gyri?

Superior and middle frontal gyri

Paracentral lobule

Parietal lobe

Lateral fissure

Insular gyrus

Posterior limb

Choroid plexus

Lateral ventricle

Frontal lobe

Putamen

Internal capsule

Anterior limb

Corpus callosum (splenium)

Cingulate gyrus Retrosplenial area

Caudate

Thalamus

Cingulate gyrus

Lateral ventricle

Corpus callosum (genu)

Occipital lobe

Interhemispheric fissure

Corpus callosum (genu)

Septum
Fornix

Choroid plexus

Merged cingulate, parieto-occipital, and calcarine sulci?

Interhemispheric fissure

4

3

14

Occipital lobe

Cingulum

5

13

Anterior complex

Dorsal complex

8

1

12

Reticular belt

Ventral complex

Posterior complex

7

6

2

Basal ganglia

Hippocampus

9

11

10

White matter

Internal capsule (anterior limb)

External capsule

Claustrum

Stria terminalis

Internal capsule (posterior limb)

Subplate

Layer I

Cortical plate

PLATE 30A
CR 235 mm
GW 26, Y16-59
Horizontal
Section 460

See detail of the brain core
in Plates 45A and B.

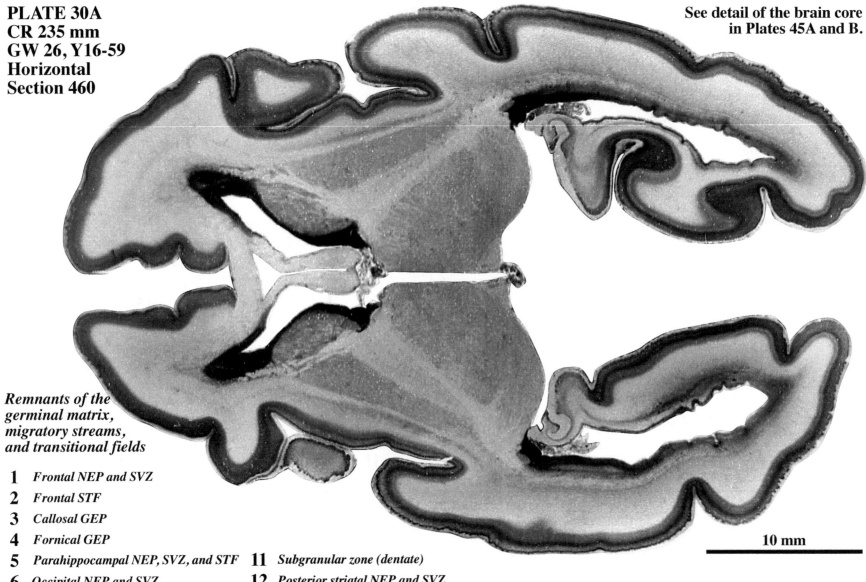

Remnants of the
germinal matrix,
migratory streams,
and transitional fields

1   *Frontal NEP and SVZ*

2   *Frontal STF*

3   *Callosal GEP*

4   *Fornical GEP*

5   *Parahippocampal NEP, SVZ, and STF*

6   *Occipital NEP and SVZ*

7   *Occipital STF*

8   *Temporal NEP and SVZ*

9   *Temporal STF*

10 *Alvear GEP*

11 *Subgranular zone (dentate)*

12 *Posterior striatal NEP and SVZ*

13 *Anterolateral striatal NEP and SVZ*

14 *Anteromedial striatal NEP and SVZ*

15 *StrionuclearGEP*

16 *Subpial granular layer (cortical)*

10 mm

GEP - Glioepithelium
NEP - Neuroepithelium
STF - Stratified transitional field
SVZ - Subventricular zone

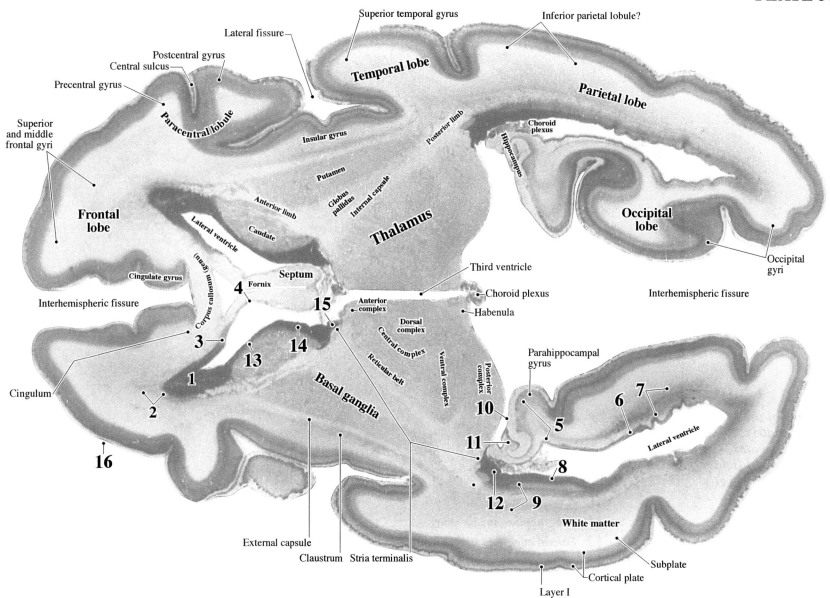

Superior temporal gyrus

Inferior parietal lobule?

Lateral fissure

Postcentral gyrus

Central sulcus

Precentral gyrus

Temporal lobe

Parietal lobe

Choroid plexus

Paracentral lobule

Superior and middle frontal gyri

Insular gyrus

Posterior limb

Hippocampus

Putamen

Globus pallidus

Internal capsule

Occipital lobe

Lateral ventricle

Caudate

Thalamus

Frontal lobe

Occipital gyri

Cingulate gyrus

Corpus callosum (genu)

Third ventricle

Interhemispheric fissure

4 *Fornix*

Septum

15

Anterior complex

Choroid plexus

Habenula

Interhemispheric fissure

Dorsal complex

3

14

Parahippocampal gyrus

Central complex

Reticular belt

Ventral complex

Posterior complex

13

Cingulum

1

Basal ganglia

10

6

7

2

5

11

16

8

12 **9**

White matter

External capsule

Lateral ventricle

Claustrum Stria terminalis

Subplate

Cortical plate

Layer I

PLATE 31A
CR 235 mm
GW 26, Y16-59
Horizontal
Section 520

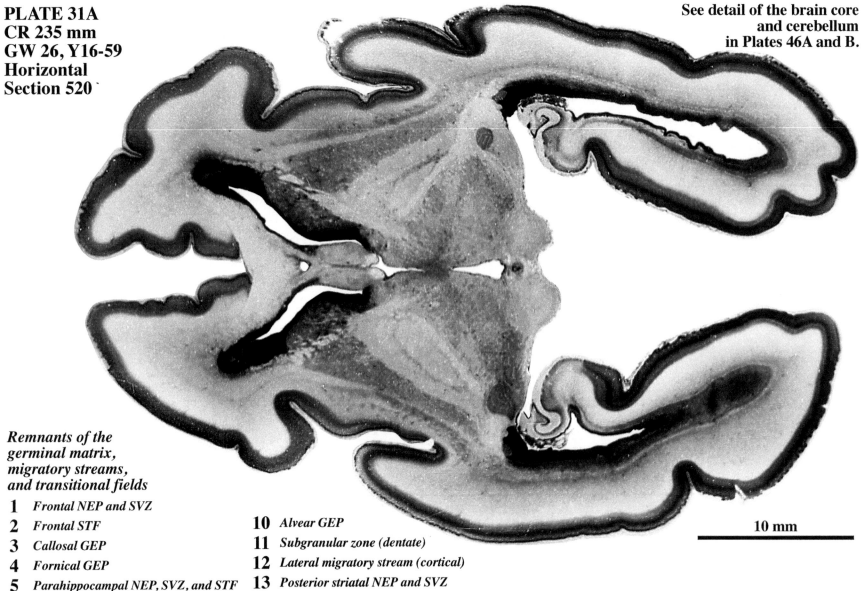

See detail of the brain core
and cerebellum
in Plates 46A and B.

10 mm

Remnants of the
germinal matrix,
migratory streams,
and transitional fields

1 *Frontal NEP and SVZ*

2 *Frontal STF*

3 *Callosal GEP*

4 *Fornical GEP*

5 *Parahippocampal NEP, SVZ, and STF*

6 *Occipital NEP and SVZ*

7 *Occipital STF*

8 *Temporal NEP and SVZ*

9 *Temporal STF*

10 *Alvear GEP*

11 *Subgranular zone (dentate)*

12 *Lateral migratory stream (cortical)*

13 *Posterior striatal NEP and SVZ*

14 *Anterolateral striatal NEP and SVZ*

15 *Anteromedial striatal NEP and SVZ*

16 *Strionuclear GEP*

17 *Subpial granular layer (cortical)*

GEP - Glioepithelium
NEP - Neuroepithelium
STF - Stratified transitional field
SVZ - Subventricular zone

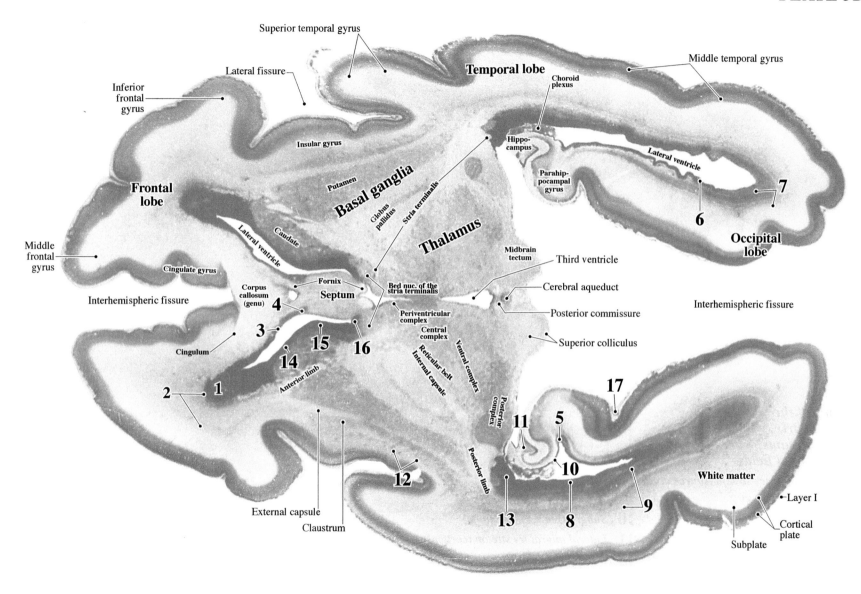

PLATE 32A
CR 235 mm
GW 26, Y16-59
Horizontal
Section 560

See detail of the brain core
and cerebellum
in Plates 47A and B.

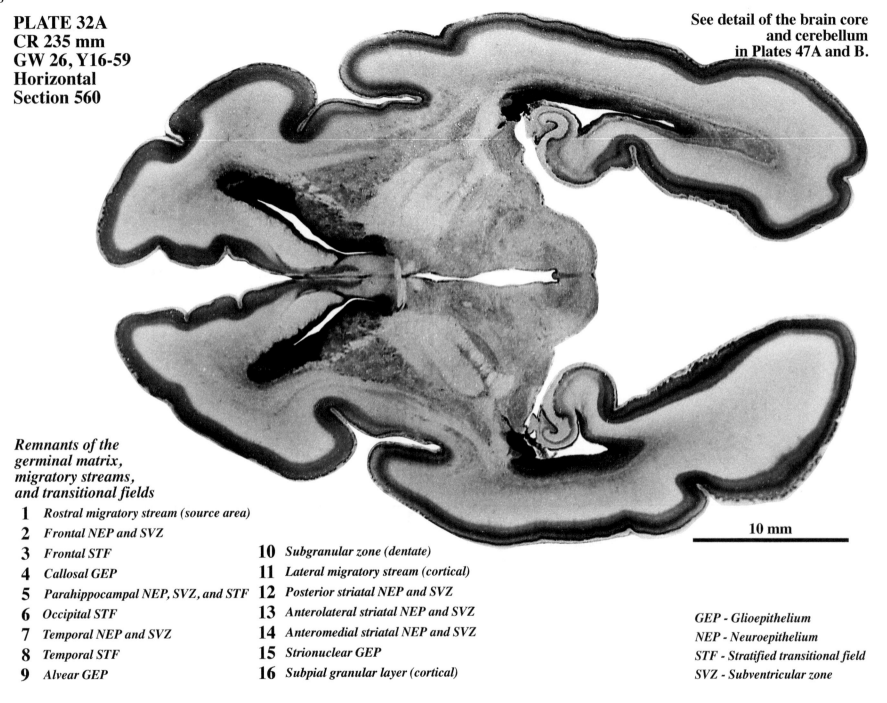

*Remnants of the
germinal matrix,
migratory streams,
and transitional fields*

1   *Rostral migratory stream (source area)*
2   *Frontal NEP and SVZ*
3   *Frontal STF*
4   *Callosal GEP*
5   *Parahippocampal NEP, SVZ, and STF*
6   *Occipital STF*
7   *Temporal NEP and SVZ*
8   *Temporal STF*
9   *Alvear GEP*

10   *Subgranular zone (dentate)*
11   *Lateral migratory stream (cortical)*
12   *Posterior striatal NEP and SVZ*
13   *Anterolateral striatal NEP and SVZ*
14   *Anteromedial striatal NEP and SVZ*
15   *Strionuclear GEP*
16   *Subpial granular layer (cortical)*

10 mm

GEP - Glioepithelium
NEP - Neuroepithelium
STF - Stratified transitional field
SVZ - Subventricular zone

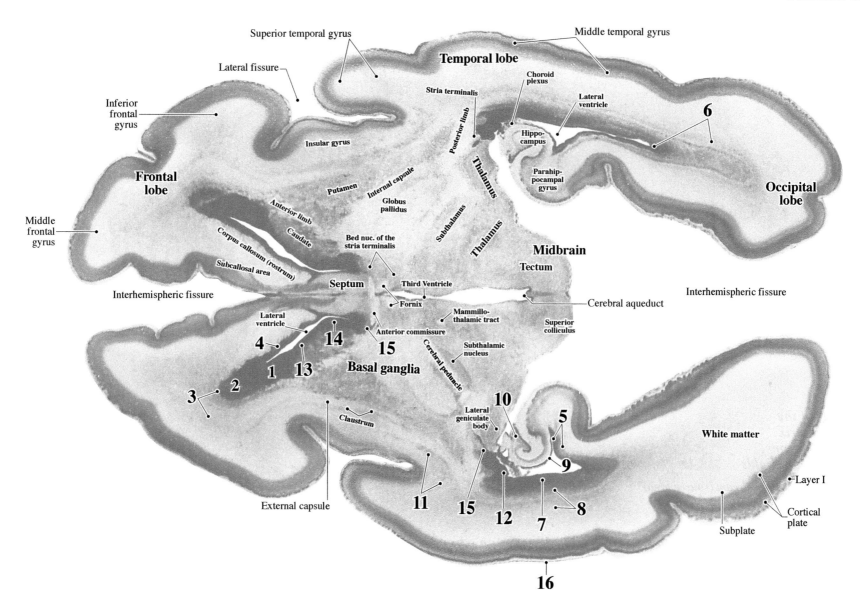

Superior temporal gyrus

Middle temporal gyrus

Temporal lobe

Lateral fissure

Choroid plexus

Stria terminalis

Lateral ventricle

Inferior frontal gyrus

6

Insular gyrus

Hippo-campus

Posterior limb

Thalamus

Parahip-pocampal gyrus

Frontal lobe

Putamen

Internal capsule

Globus pallidus

Occipital lobe

Anterior limb

Subthalamus

Thalamus

Middle frontal gyrus

Caudate

Bed nuc. of the stria terminalis

Thalamus

Midbrain

Corpus callosum (rostrum)

Tectum

Subcallosal area

Septum

Third Ventricle

Interhemispheric fissure

Cerebral aqueduct

Interhemispheric fissure

Fornix

Mammillo-thalamic tract

Lateral ventricle

Anterior commissure

Superior colliculus

4

14

Subthalamic nucleus

15

Cerebral peduncle

1

13

Basal ganglia

2

3

Claustrum

Lateral geniculate body

10

5

White matter

9

External capsule

11

15

12

8

Layer I

7

Cortical plate

16

Subplate

PLATE 33A
CR 235 mm
GW 26, Y16-59
Horizontal
Section 620

See detail of the brain core and cerebellum
in Plates 48A and B.

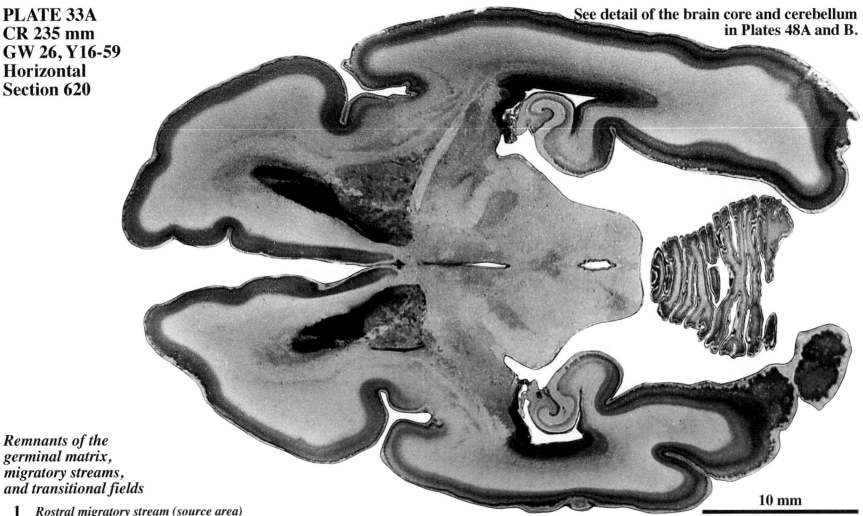

10 mm

Remnants of the
germinal matrix,
migratory streams,
and transitional fields

1 *Rostral migratory stream (source area)*
2 *Frontal NEP and SVZ*
3 *Frontal STF*
4 *Parahippocampal NEP, SVZ, and STF*
5 *Temporal NEP and SVZ*
6 *Temporal STF*
7 *Alvear GEP*
8 *Subgranular zone (dentate)*
9 *Lateral migratory stream (cortical)*

10 *Posterior striatal NEP and SVZ*
11 *Accumbent NEP (intermingled with the rostral migratory stream)*
12 *Diencephalic (hypothalamic) G/EP*
13 *Mesencephalic G/EP*
14 *External germinal layer (cerebellar)*
15 *Subpial granular layer (cortical)*

GEP - Glioepithelium
G/EP - Glioepithelium/ependyma
NEP - Neuroepithelium
STF - Stratified transitional field
SVZ - Subventricular zone

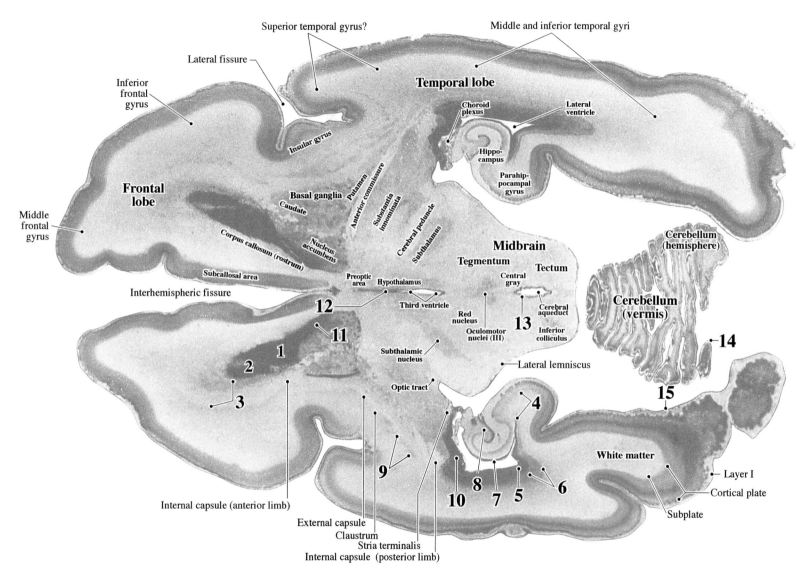

Superior temporal gyrus?

Middle and inferior temporal gyri

Lateral fissure

Temporal lobe

Inferior
frontal
gyrus

Choroid
plexus

Lateral
ventricle

Insular gyrus

Hippo-
campus

Parahip-
pocampal
gyrus

Frontal
lobe

Basal ganglia

Putamen

Anterior commissure

Substantia inmominata

Caudate

Cerebral peduncle

Midbrain

Cerebellum
(hemisphere)

Middle
frontal
gyrus

Corpus callosum (rostrum)

Nucleus
accumbens

Subthalamus

Tegmentum

Tectum

Central
gray

Subcallosal area

Preoptic
area

Hypothalamus

Cerebral
aqueduct

Cerebellum
(vermis)

Interhemispheric fissure

Third ventricle

12

Red
nucleus

13

11

Oculomotor
nuclei (III)

Inferior
colliculus

1

2

Subthalamic
nucleus

14

3

Lateral lemniscus

Optic tract

4

15

White matter

9

8

10

7

5

6

Layer I

Internal capsule (anterior limb)

Cortical plate

External capsule

Subplate

Claustrum

Stria terminalis

Internal capsule (posterior limb)

PLATE 34A
CR 235 mm
GW 26, Y16-59
Horizontal
Section 660

See detail of the brain core
and cerebellum
in Plates 49A and B.

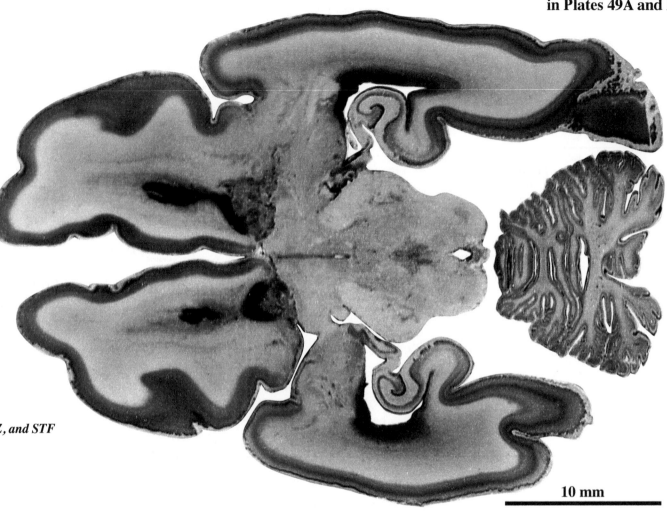

Remnants of the
germinal matrix,
migratory streams,
and transitional fields

1 *Rostral migratory stream*
2 *Frontal NEP and SVZ*
3 *Frontal STF*
4 *Parahippocampal NEP, SVZ, and STF*
5 *Temporal NEP and SVZ*
6 *Temporal STF*
7 *Alvear GEP*
8 *Subgranular zone (dentate)*
9 *Lateral migratory stream (cortical)*
10 *Amygdaloid G/EP*
11 *Diencephalic (hypothalamic) G/EP*
12 *Mesencephalic G/EP*
13 *External germinal layer (cerebellar)*
14 *Subpial granular layer (cortical)*

10 mm

GEP - Glioepithelium
G/EP - Glioepithelium/ependyma
NEP - Neuroepithelium
STF - Stratified transitional field
SVZ - Subventricular zone

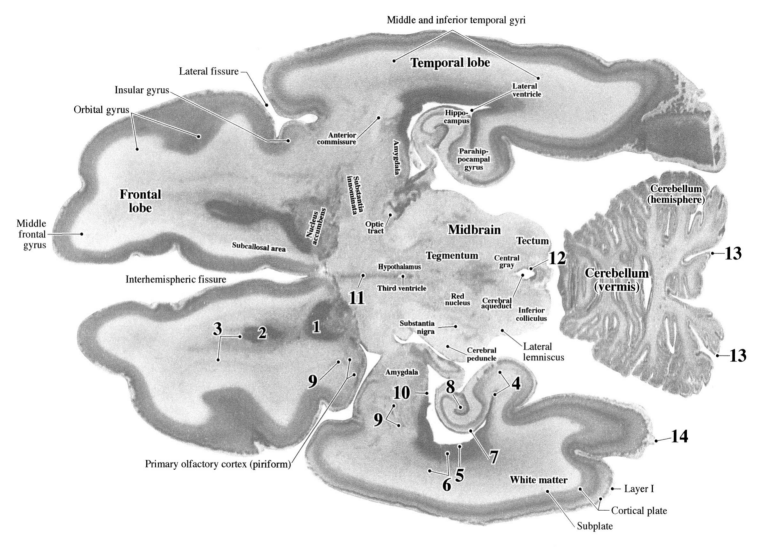

Middle and inferior temporal gyri

Temporal lobe

Lateral fissure

Insular gyrus

Orbital gyrus

Lateral ventricle

Hippo- campus

Anterior commissure

Amygdala

Parahip- pocampal gyrus

Substantia innominata

Frontal lobe

Nucleus accumbens

Optic tract

Midbrain

Tectum

Cerebellum (hemisphere)

Middle frontal gyrus

Subcallosal area

Tegmentum

Central gray

12

Cerebellum (vermis)

13

Hypothalamus

Third ventricle

Red nucleus

Cerebral aqueduct

Interhemispheric fissure

11

Substantia nigra

Inferior colliculus

3 **2** **1**

Cerebral peduncle

Lateral lemniscus

9

Amygdala

4

13

9

10

8

7

14

Primary olfactory cortex (piriform)

9

5

6

White matter

Layer I

Cortical plate

Subplate

74

PLATE 35A
CR 235 mm
GW 26, Y16-59
Horizontal
Section 700

See detail of the brain core
and cerebellum
in Plates 50A and B.

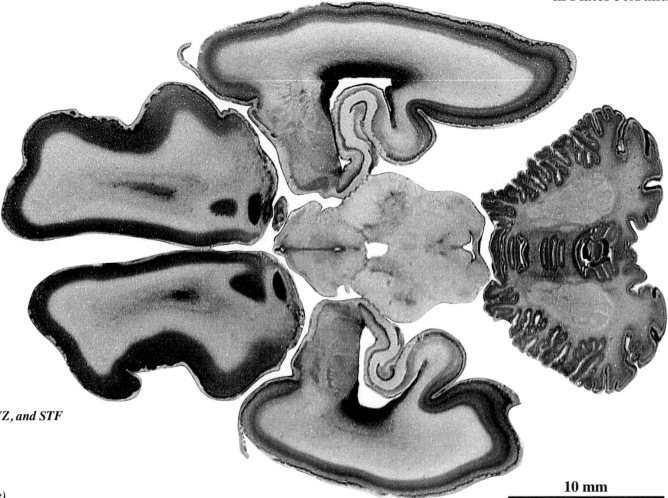

Remnants of the
germinal matrix,
migratory streams,
and transitional fields

1 *Rostral migratory stream*

2 *Frontal NEP and SVZ*

3 *Frontal STF*

4 *Parahippocampal NEP, SVZ, and STF*

5 *Temporal NEP and SVZ*

6 *Temporal STF*

7 *Alvear GEP*

8 *Subgranular zone (dentate)*

9 *Lateral migratory stream (cortical)*

10 *Amygdaloid G/EP*

11 *Diencephalic (hypothalamic) G/EP*

12 *Mesencephalic G/EP*

13 *External germinal layer (cerebellar)*

14 *Subpial granular layer (cortical)*

GEP - Glioepithelium
G/EP - Glioepithelium/ependyma
NEP - Neuroepithelium
STF - Stratified transitional field
SVZ - Subventricular zone

10 mm

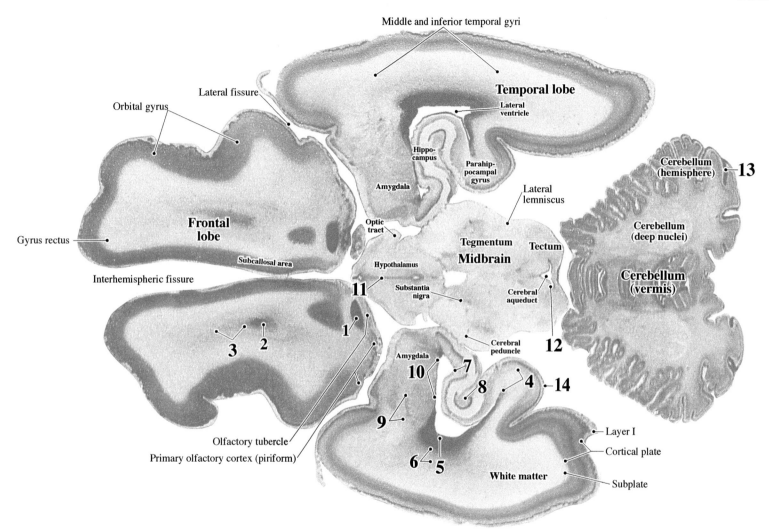

Middle and inferior temporal gyri

Lateral fissure

Orbital gyrus

Temporal lobe

Lateral ventricle

Hippo-campus

Parahip-pocampal gyrus

Amygdala

Cerebellum (hemisphere) —**13**

Lateral lemniscus

Frontal lobe

Optic tract

Cerebellum (deep nuclei)

Gyrus rectus

Tegmentum
Midbrain

Tectum

Cerebellum (vermis)

Subcallosal area

Hypothalamus

11

Interhemispheric fissure

Substantia nigra

Cerebral aqueduct

1

3 **2**

Cerebral peduncle

12

Amygdala

7

10

8 **4** —**14**

Olfactory tubercle

9

Layer I

Primary olfactory cortex (piriform)

Cortical plate

6 **5**

White matter

Subplate

PLATE 36A
CR 235 mm
GW 26, Y16-59
Horizontal
Section 740

See detail of the brain core
and cerebellum
in Plates 51A and B.

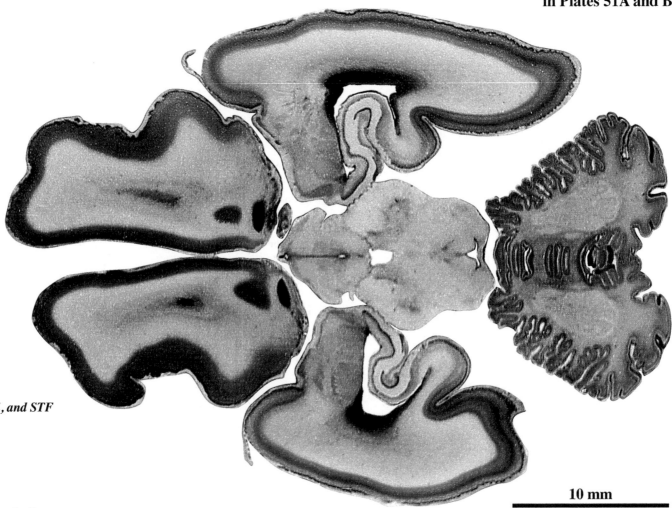

Remnants of the
germinal matrix,
migratory streams,
and transitional fields

1 *Rostral migratory stream*

2 *Frontal STF*

3 *Parahippocampal NEP, SVZ, and STF*

4 *Temporal NEP and SVZ*

5 *Temporal STF*

6 *Alvear GEP*

7 *Subgranular zone (dentate)*

8 *Lateral migratory stream (cortical)*

9 *Amygdaloid G/EP*

10 *Diencephalic (hypothalamic) G/EP*

11 *Pontine G/EP*

12 *External germinal layer (cerebellar)*

13 *Subpial granular layer (cortical)*

GEP - Glioepithelium
G/EP - Glioepithelium/ependyma
NEP - Neuroepithelium
STF - Stratified transitional field
SVZ - Subventricular zone

10 mm

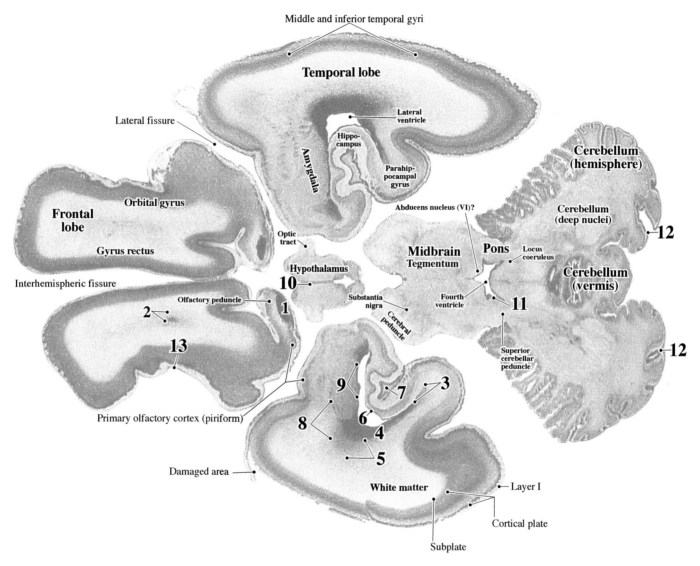

Middle and inferior temporal gyri

Temporal lobe

Lateral fissure

Lateral ventricle

Hippo-campus

Amygdala

Parahip-pocampal gyrus

Cerebellum (hemisphere)

Cerebellum (deep nuclei)

Abducens nucleus (VI)?

Orbital gyrus

Frontal lobe

Optic tract

Midbrain Tegmentum

Pons

Locus coeruleus

12

Gyrus rectus

Hypothalamus

Cerebellum (vermis)

Interhemispheric fissure

10

Substantia nigra

Fourth ventricle

Olfactory peduncle

1

Cerebral peduncle

11

2

13

Superior cerebellar peduncle

12

9

7

3

Primary olfactory cortex (piriform)

8

6

4

5

Damaged area

White matter

Layer I

Cortical plate

Subplate

PLATE 37A
CR 235 mm
GW 26, Y16-59
Horizontal
Section 780

See detail of the brain core
and cerebellum
in Plates 52A and B.

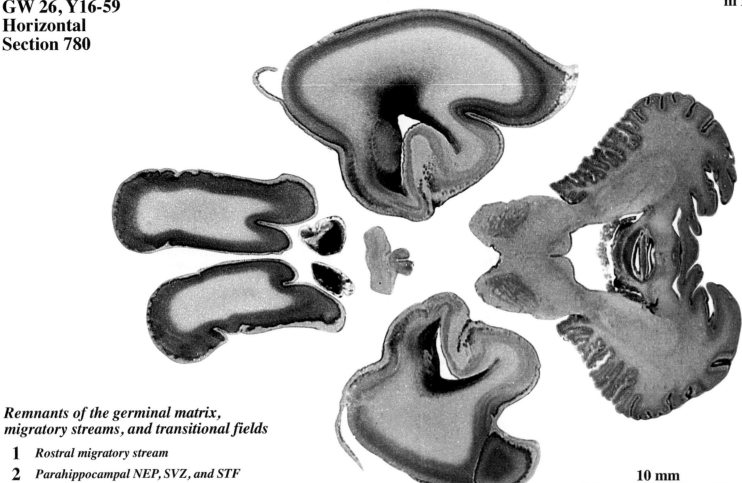

Remnants of the germinal matrix,
migratory streams, and transitional fields

1 *Rostral migratory stream*

2 *Parahippocampal NEP, SVZ, and STF*

3 *Temporal NEP, SVZ, and STF*

4 *Alvear GEP*

5 *Lateral migratory stream (cortical)*

6 *Amygdaloid G/EP*

7 *Pontine G/EP*

8 *External germinal layer (cerebellar)*

9 *Subpial granular layer (cortical)*

GEP - Glioepithelium
G/EP - Glioepithelium/ependyma
NEP - Neuroepithelium
STF - Stratified transitional field
SVZ - Subventricular zone

10 mm

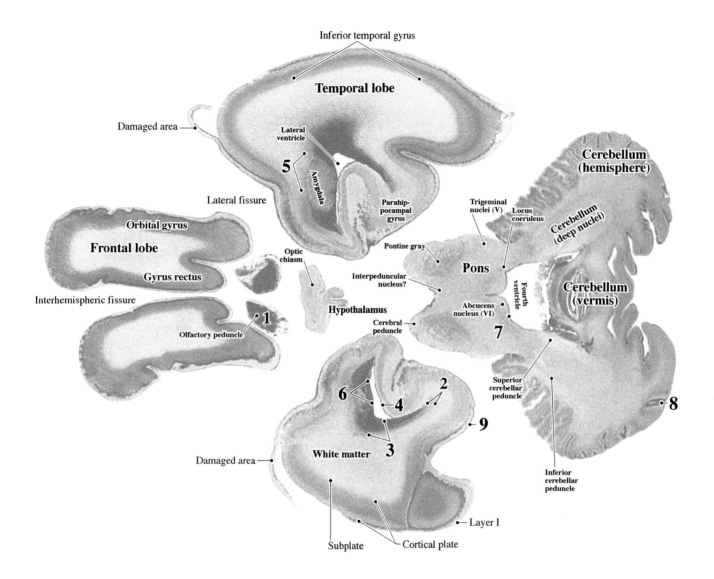

Inferior temporal gyrus

Temporal lobe

Damaged area

Lateral ventricle

5

Amygdala

Lateral fissure

Parahip-pocampal gyrus

Orbital gyrus

Frontal lobe

Optic chiasm

Gyrus rectus

Interhemispheric fissure

1

Olfactory peduncle

Pontine gray

Interpeduncular nucleus?

Hypothalamus

Cerebral peduncle

Trigeminal nuclei (V)

Locus coeruleus

Pons

Abcucens nucleus (VI)

Fourth ventricle

Cerebellum (hemisphere)

Cerebellum (deep nuclei)

Cerebellum (vermis)

7

Superior cerebellar peduncle

6

2

4

9

3

White matter

8

Inferior cerebellar peduncle

Damaged area

Subplate

Cortical plate

Layer I

PLATE 38A
CR 235 mm
GW 26, Y16-59
Horizontal
Section 820

See detail of the brain core
and cerebellum
in Plates 53A and B.

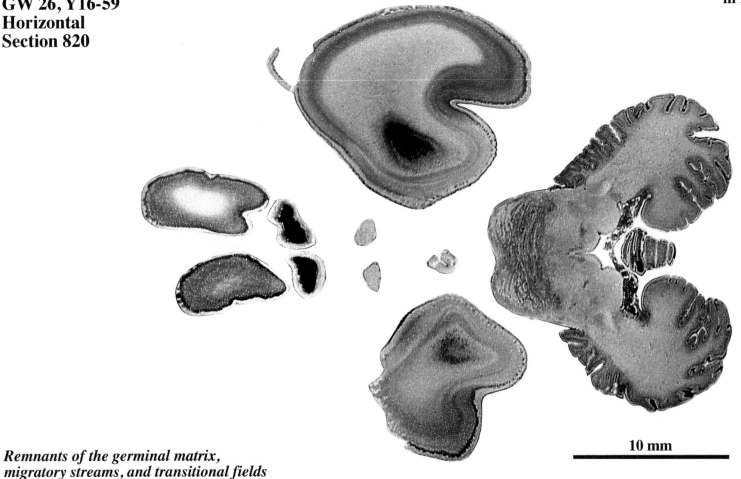

10 mm

Remnants of the germinal matrix,
migratory streams, and transitional fields

1 *Rostral migratory stream*

2 *Parahippocampal NEP, SVZ, and STF*

3 *Temporal NEP, SVZ, and STF*

4 *Amygdaloid G/EP*

5 *Medullary G/EP*

6 *External germinal layer (cerebellar)*

7 *Subpial granular layer (cortical)*

G/EP - Glioepithelium/ependyma
NEP - Neuroepithelium
STF - Stratified transitional field
SVZ - Subventricular zone

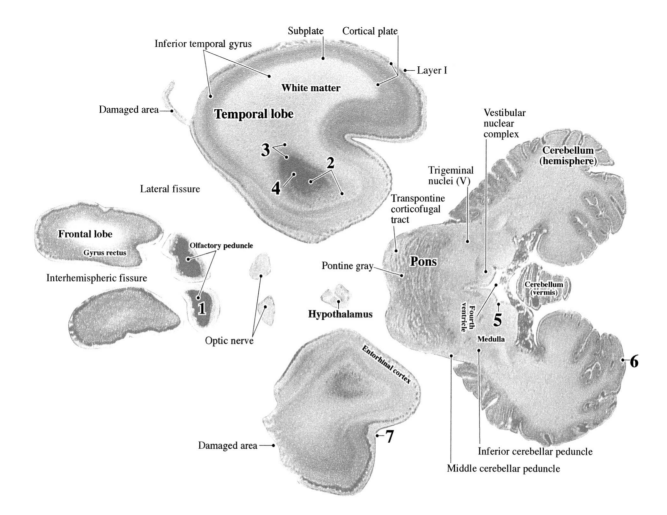

Subplate
Cortical plate
Inferior temporal gyrus
Layer I
White matter
Damaged area
Temporal lobe
3
2
Lateral fissure
4
Frontal lobe
Gyrus rectus
Olfactory peduncle
Interhemispheric fissure
1
Hypothalamus
Optic nerve
Pontine gray
Vestibular
nuclear
complex
**Cerebellum
(hemisphere)**
Trigeminal
nuclei (V)
Transpontine
corticofugal
tract
Pons
Fourth
ventricle
**Cerebellum
(vermis)**
5
Medulla
6
Entorhinal cortex
7
Damaged area
Inferior cerebellar peduncle
Middle cerebellar peduncle

PLATE 39A
CR 235 mm
GW 26, Y16-59
Horizontal
Section 860

See detail of the brain core
and cerebellum
in Plates 54A and B.

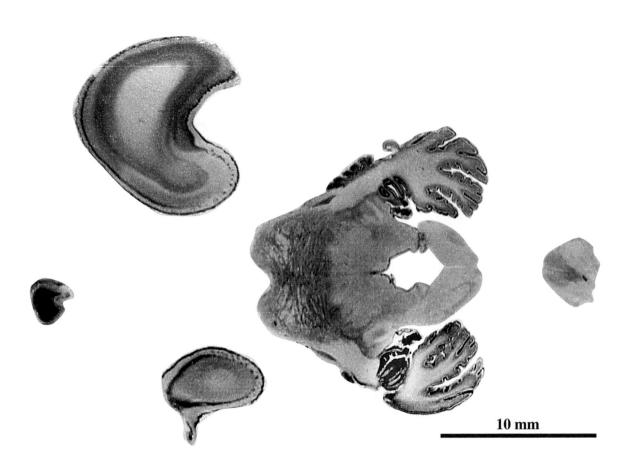

10 mm

Remnants of the germinal matrix,
migratory streams, and transitional fields

1 *Rostral migratory stream*

2 *Medullary glioepithelium/ependyma*

3 *External germinal layer (cerebellar)*

4 *Subpial granular layer (cortical)*

5 *Dorsal funicular myelination gliosis*

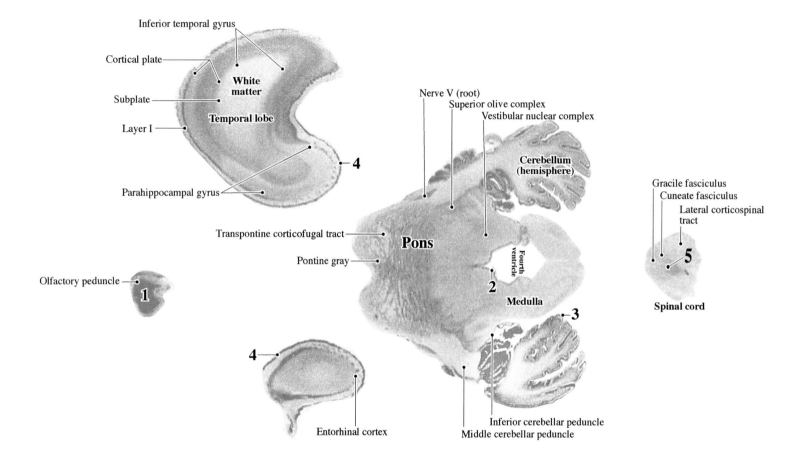

Inferior temporal gyrus

Cortical plate

White matter

Subplate

Temporal lobe

Layer I

Parahippocampal gyrus

Nerve V (root)

Superior olive complex

Vestibular nuclear complex

Cerebellum (hemisphere)

Gracile fasciculus

Cuneate fasciculus

Lateral corticospinal tract

4

Transpontine corticofugal tract

Pons

Pontine gray

Fourth ventricle

5

Olfactory peduncle

1

2

Medulla

3

Spinal cord

4

Inferior cerebellar peduncle

Middle cerebellar peduncle

Entorhinal cortex

PLATE 40A
CR 235 mm
GW 26, Y16-59
Horizontal
Section 880

See detail of the brain core
and cerebellum
in Plates 55A and B.

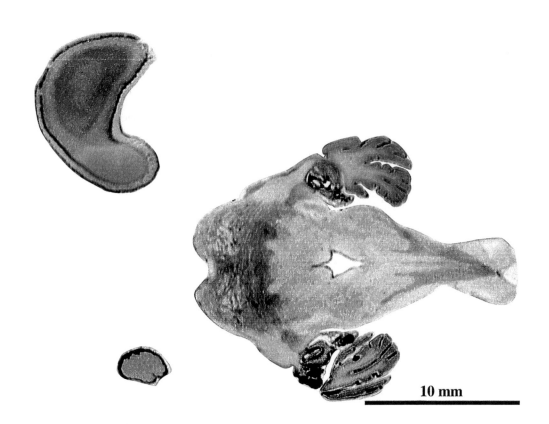

10 mm

Remnants of the germinal matrix,
migratory streams, and transitional fields

1 *Medullary glioepithelium/ependyma*

2 *External germinal layer (cerebellar)*

3 *Subpial granular layer (cortical)*

4 *Dorsal funicular myelination gliosis*

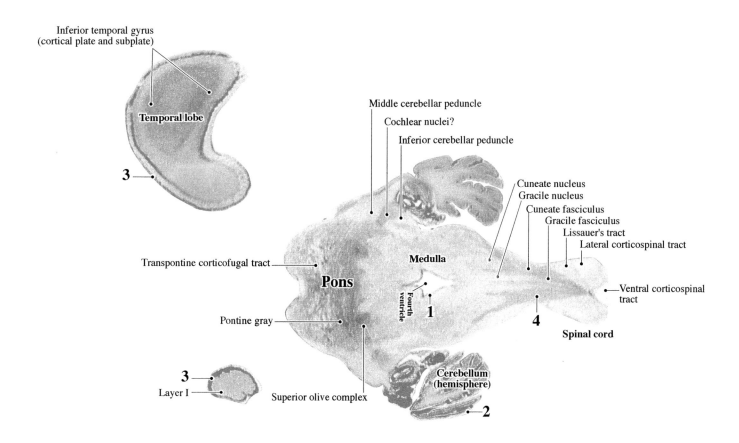

Inferior temporal gyrus
(cortical plate and subplate)

Temporal lobe

3

Middle cerebellar peduncle

Cochlear nuclei?

Inferior cerebellar peduncle

Cuneate nucleus
Gracile nucleus
Cuneate fasciculus
Gracile fasciculus
Lissauer's tract
Lateral corticospinal tract

Medulla

Transpontine corticofugal tract

Pons

Fourth
ventricle
1

Ventral corticospinal
tract

Pontine gray

4

Spinal cord

3

**Cerebellum
(hemisphere)**

Layer I

Superior olive complex

2

86

See detail of the brain core
and cerebellum
in Plates 56A and B.

PLATE 41A
CR 235 mm
GW 26, Y16-59
Horizontal
Section 900

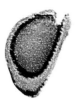

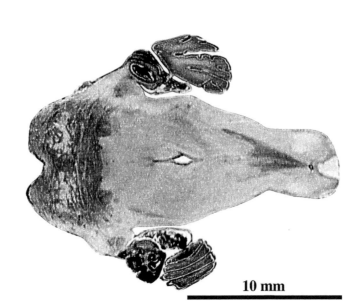

10 mm

Remnants of the germinal matrix,
migratory streams, and transitional fields

1 *Medullary glioepithelium/ependyma*

2 *External germinal layer (cerebellar)*

3 *Subpial granular layer (cortical)*

4 *Dorsal funicular myelination gliosis*

5 *Ventral funicular myelination gliosis*

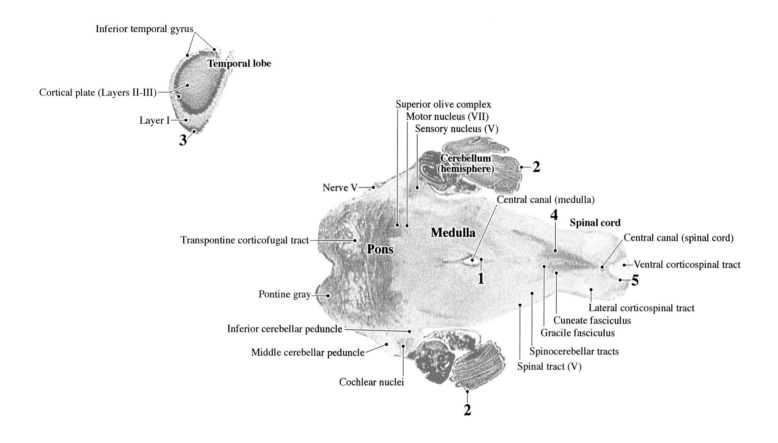

Inferior temporal gyrus

Temporal lobe

Cortical plate (Layers II-III)

Layer I

3

Superior olive complex
Motor nucleus (VII)
Sensory nucleus (V)

**Cerebellum
(hemisphere)**

2

Nerve V

Central canal (medulla)

4

Spinal cord

Medulla

Central canal (spinal cord)

Transpontine corticofugal tract

Pons

Ventral corticospinal tract

1

5

Pontine gray

Lateral corticospinal tract

Inferior cerebellar peduncle

Cuneate fasciculus

Middle cerebellar peduncle

Gracile fasciculus

Spinocerebellar tracts

Cochlear nuclei

Spinal tract (V)

2

PLATE 42A
CR 235 mm
GW 26, Y16-59
Horizontal
Section 940

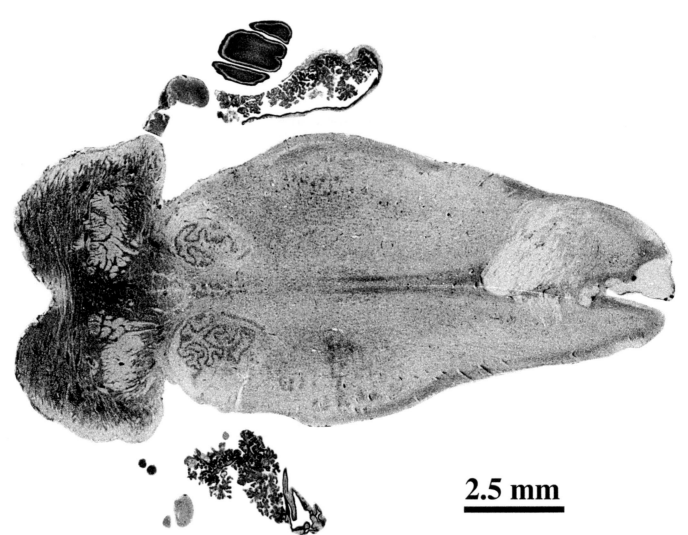

2.5 mm

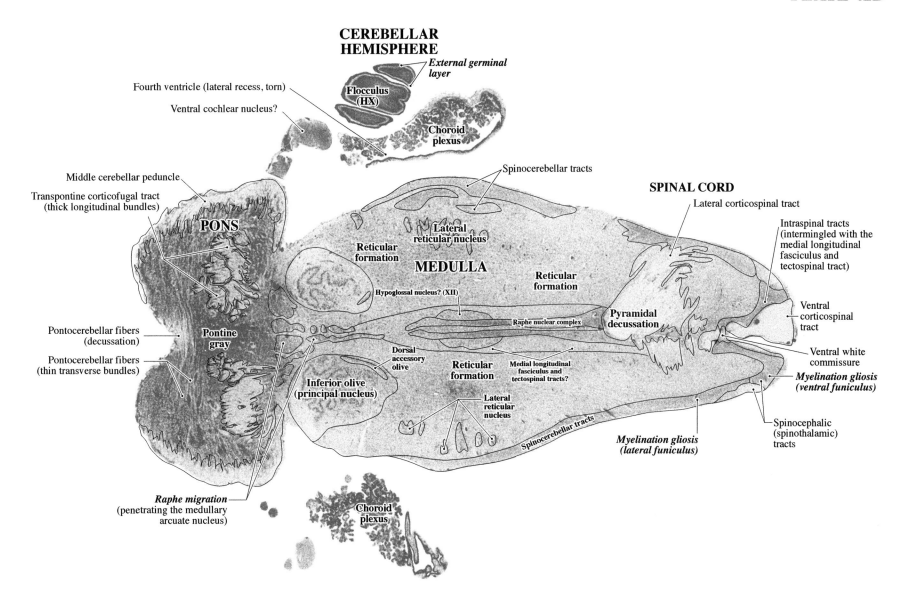

CEREBELLAR HEMISPHERE

External germinal layer

Fourth ventricle (lateral recess, torn)

Flocculus (HX)

Ventral cochlear nucleus?

Choroid plexus

Spinocerebellar tracts

SPINAL CORD

Middle cerebellar peduncle

Transpontine corticofugal tract (thick longitudinal bundles)

PONS

Lateral corticospinal tract

Intraspinal tracts (intermingled with the medial longitudinal fasciculus and tectospinal tract)

Lateral reticular nucleus

Reticular formation

MEDULLA

Reticular formation

Hypoglossal nucleus? (XII)

Raphe nuclear complex

Pyramidal decussation

Pontocerebellar fibers (decussation)

Pontine gray

Ventral corticospinal tract

Dorsal accessory olive

Reticular formation

Medial longitudinal fasciculus and tectospinal tracts?

Pontocerebellar fibers (thin transverse bundles)

Ventral white commissure

Inferior olive (principal nucleus)

Myelination gliosis (ventral funiculus)

Lateral reticular nucleus

Spinocerebellar tracts

Myelination gliosis (lateral funiculus)

Spinocephalic (spinothalamic) tracts

Raphe migration (penetrating the medullary arcuate nucleus)

Choroid plexus

Germinal and transitional structures in *italics*

90

**PLATE 43A
CR 235 mm
GW 26, Y16-59
Horizontal
Section 960**

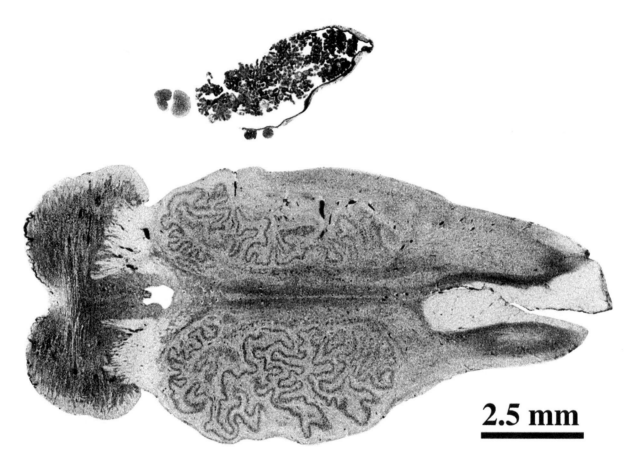

2.5 mm

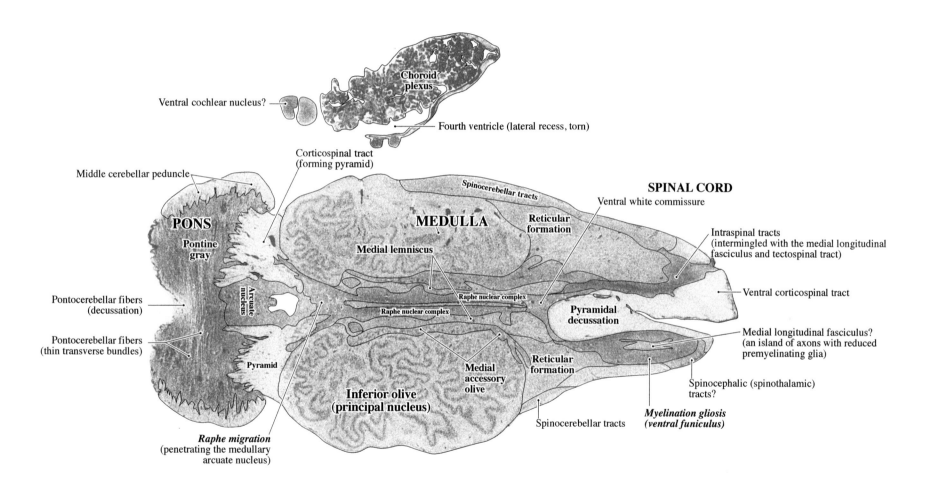

Choroid plexus

Ventral cochlear nucleus?

Fourth ventricle (lateral recess, torn)

Corticospinal tract
(forming pyramid)

Middle cerebellar peduncle

Spinocerebellar tracts

SPINAL CORD
Ventral white commissure

PONS

MEDULLA

Reticular
formation

Pontine
gray

Intraspinal tracts
(intermingled with the medial longitudinal
fasciculus and tectospinal tract)

Medial lemniscus

Pontocerebellar fibers
(decussation)

Arcuate
nucleus

Raphe nuclear complex

Raphe nuclear complex

Ventral corticospinal tract

Pyramidal
decussation

Pontocerebellar fibers
(thin transverse bundles)

Medial longitudinal fasciculus?
(an island of axons with reduced
premyelinating glia)

Pyramid

Medial
accessory
olive

Reticular
formation

Spinocephalic (spinothalamic)
tracts?

**Inferior olive
(principal nucleus)**

Spinocerebellar tracts

*Myelination gliosis
(ventral funiculus)*

Raphe migration
(penetrating the medullary
arcuate nucleus)

**Germinal and transitional
structures in *italics***

PLATE 44A, CR 235 mm, GW 26, Y16-59
Horizontal, Section 400

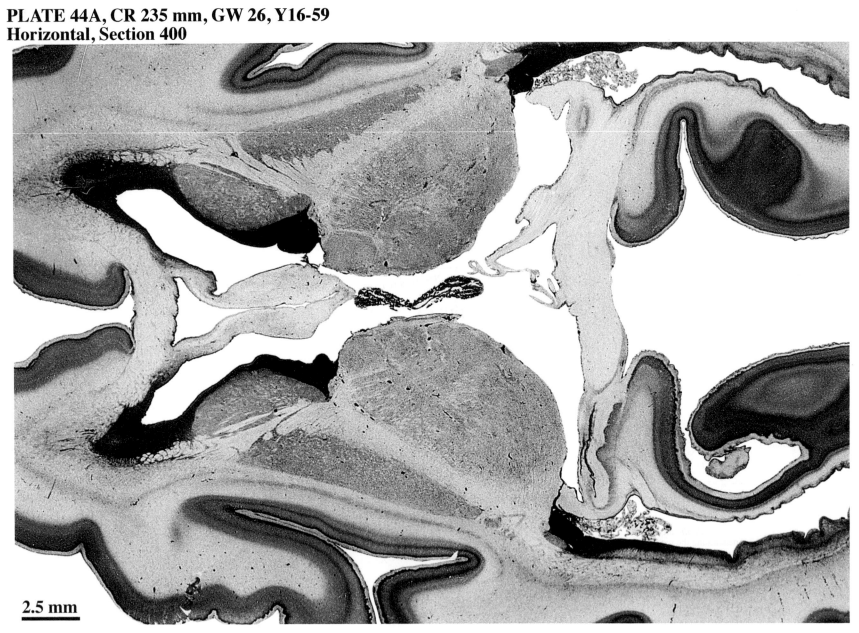

2.5 mm

See the entire Section 400 in Plate 29.

93

PLATE 44B

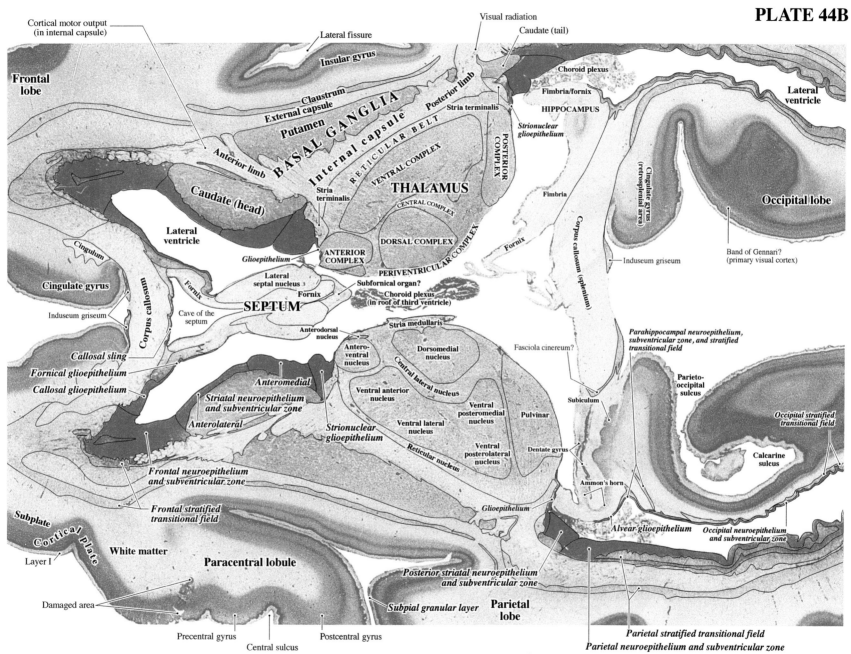

Cortical motor output (in internal capsule)
Lateral fissure
Visual radiation
Caudate (tail)

Insular gyrus
Choroid plexus

Frontal lobe
Claustrum
External capsule
Putamen
BASAL GANGLIA
Fimbria/fornix
HIPPOCAMPUS
Lateral ventricle

Posterior limb
Stria terminalis
Strionuclear glioepithelium

Anterior limb
Internal capsule
RETICULAR BELT
VENTRAL COMPLEX
POSTERIOR COMPLEX

Caudate (head)
Stria terminalis
THALAMUS
Fimbria
Occipital lobe

CENTRAL COMPLEX

Lateral ventricle
Glioepithelium
ANTERIOR COMPLEX
DORSAL COMPLEX
PERIVENTRICULAR COMPLEX
Fornix
Corpus callosum (splenium)
Cingulate gyrus (retrosplenial area)

Cingulum

Cingulate gyrus
Fornix
Lateral septal nucleus
Subfornical organ?
Choroid plexus (in roof of third ventricle)
Band of Gennari? (primary visual cortex)

Corpus callosum
Fornix
Fornix
SEPTUM
Induseum griseum

Induseum griseum
Cave of the septum
Stria medullaris
Fasciola cinereum?
Parahippocampal neuroepithelium, subventricular zone, and stratified transitional field

Anterodorsal nucleus
Dorsomedial nucleus

Callosal sling
Fornical glioepithelium
Callosal glioepithelium
Antero-ventral nucleus
Central lateral nucleus
Parieto-occipital sulcus

Anteromedial
Ventral anterior nucleus
Ventral posteromedial nucleus
Pulvinar
Subiculum
Occipital stratified transitional field

Striatal neuroepithelium and subventricular zone
Anterolateral
Strionuclear glioepithelium
Ventral lateral nucleus
Ventral posterolateral nucleus
Dentate gyrus
Calcarine sulcus

Reticular nucleus
Ammon's horn

Frontal neuroepithelium and subventricular zone
Glioepithelium
Alvear glioepithelium
Occipital neuroepithelium and subventricular zone

Frontal stratified transitional field

Subplate
White matter
Paracentral lobule
Posterior striatal neuroepithelium and subventricular zone

Cortical Plate
Layer I
Subpial granular layer
Parietal lobe

Damaged area
Precentral gyrus
Central sulcus
Postcentral gyrus
Parietal stratified transitional field
Parietal neuroepithelium and subventricular zone

Germinal and transitional structures in *italics*

PLATE 45A
CR 235 mm
GW 26, Y16-59
Horizontal
Section 460

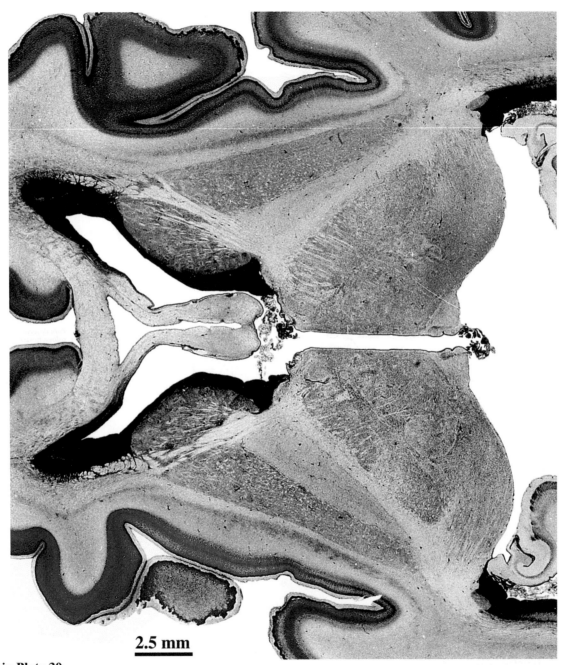

2.5 mm

See the entire Section 460 in Plate 30.

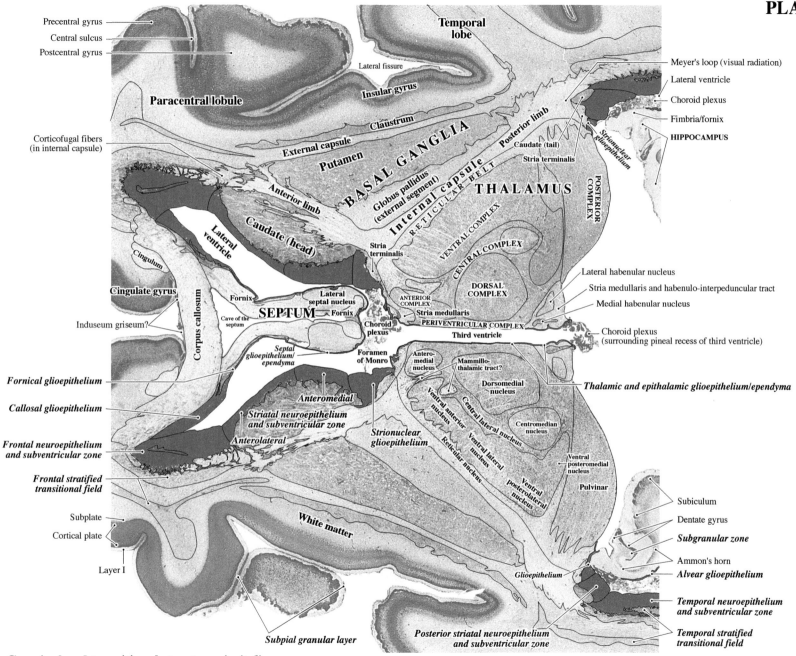

Precentral gyrus
Central sulcus
Postcentral gyrus
Lateral fissure
Temporal lobe
Meyer's loop (visual radiation)
Lateral ventricle
Choroid plexus
Paracentral lobule
Insular gyrus
Claustrum
Fimbria/fornix
Strionuclear glioepithelium
HIPPOCAMPUS
Corticofugal fibers (in internal capsule)
External capsule
Putamen
BASAL GANGLIA
Posterior limb
Caudate (tail)
Stria terminalis
Anterior limb
Globus pallidus (external segment)
Internal capsule
RETICULAR BELT
THALAMUS
POSTERIOR COMPLEX
Caudate (head)
Lateral ventricle
Cingulum
VENTRAL COMPLEX
CENTRAL COMPLEX
Stria terminalis
Cingulate gyrus
Fornix
Lateral septal nucleus
ANTERIOR COMPLEX
DORSAL COMPLEX
Lateral habenular nucleus
Stria medullaris and habenulo-interpeduncular tract
Medial habenular nucleus
Cave of the septum
SEPTUM
Fornix
Stria medullaris
PERIVENTRICULAR COMPLEX
Induseum griseum?
Corpus callosum
Choroid plexus
Third ventricle
Choroid plexus (surrounding pineal recess of third ventricle)
Septal glioepithelium/ ependyma
Foramen of Monro
Antero-medial nucleus
Mammillo-thalamic tract?
Fornical glioepithelium
Anteromedial
Dorsomedial nucleus
Ventral anterior nucleus
Central lateral nucleus
Thalamic and epithalamic glioepithelium/ependyma
Callosal glioepithelium
Striatal neuroepithelium and subventricular zone
Strionuclear glioepithelium
Centromedian nucleus
Frontal neuroepithelium and subventricular zone
Anterolateral
Ventral lateral nucleus
Reticular nucleus
Ventral posterolateral nucleus
Ventral posteromedial nucleus
Frontal stratified transitional field
Pulvinar
Subiculum
Subplate
Cortical plate
White matter
Dentate gyrus
Subgranular zone
Layer I
Glioepithelium
Ammon's horn
Alvear glioepithelium
Temporal neuroepithelium and subventricular zone
Subpial granular layer
Posterior striatal neuroepithelium and subventricular zone
Temporal stratified transitional field

Germinal and transitional structures in *italics*

PLATE 46A
CR 235 mm
GW 26, Y16-59
Horizontal
Section 520

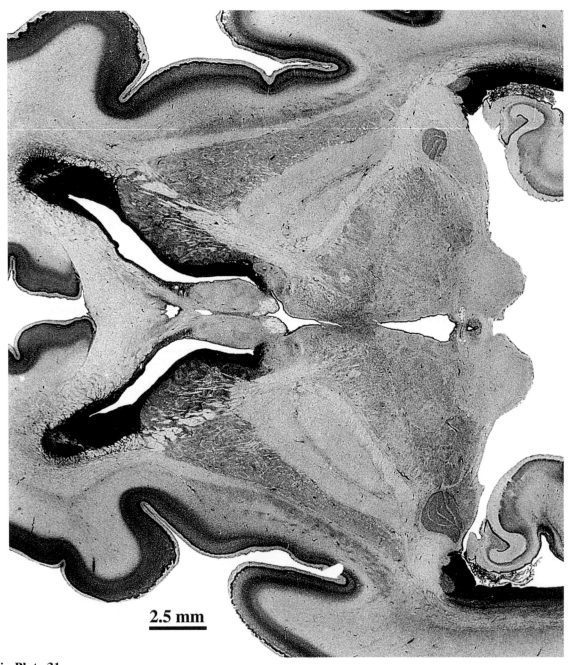

2.5 mm

See the entire Section 520 in Plate 31.

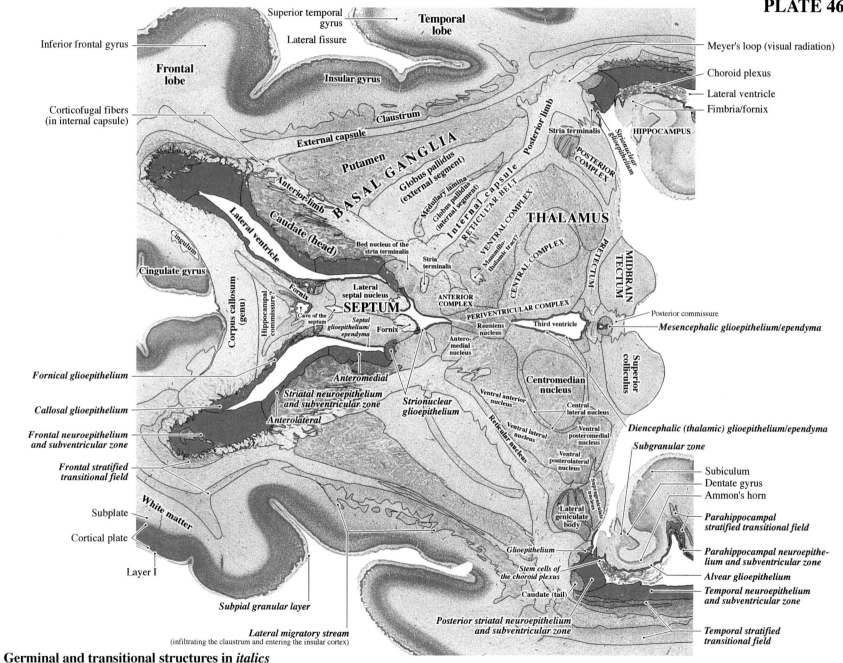

Superior temporal gyrus

Temporal lobe

Lateral fissure

Inferior frontal gyrus

Meyer's loop (visual radiation)

Frontal lobe

Insular gyrus

Choroid plexus

Lateral ventricle

Fimbria/fornix

Corticofugal fibers (in internal capsule)

Claustrum

External capsule

Putamen

Globus pallidus (external segment)

Medullary lamina

Globus pallidus (internal segment)

Internal capsule

Posterior limb

Stria terminalis

HIPPOCAMPUS

Strionuclear glioepithelium

POSTERIOR COMPLEX

BASAL GANGLIA

RETICULAR BELT

VENTRAL COMPLEX

THALAMUS

Anterior limb

Caudate (head)

Bed nucleus of the stria terminalis

Stria terminalis

Mammillo-thalamic tract?

CENTRAL COMPLEX

PRETECTUM

MIDBRAIN TECTUM

Cingulum

Lateral ventricle

Cingulate gyrus

Cingulum

Fornix

Lateral septal nucleus

SEPTUM

ANTERIOR COMPLEX

PERIVENTRICULAR COMPLEX

Posterior commissure

Hippocampal commissure?

Cave of the septum

Septal glioepithelium/ ependyma

Fornix

Reuniens nucleus

Third ventricle

Mesencephalic glioepithelium/ependyma

Corpus callosum (genu)

Antero-medial nucleus

Superior colliculus

Fornical glioepithelium

Anteromedial

Centromedian nucleus

Callosal glioepithelium

Striatal neuroepithelium and subventricular zone

Strionuclear glioepithelium

Ventral anterior nucleus

Central lateral nucleus

Diencephalic (thalamic) glioepithelium/ependyma

Frontal neuroepithelium and subventricular zone

Anterolateral

Ventral lateral nucleus

Ventral posteromedial nucleus

Subgranular zone

Reticular nucleus

Frontal stratified transitional field

Ventral posterolateral nucleus

Subiculum

Dentate gyrus

Ammon's horn

Subplate

White matter

Suprageniculate nucleus

Lateral geniculate body

Parahippocampal stratified transitional field

Cortical plate

Parahippocampal neuroepithe-lium and subventricular zone

Layer I

Glioepithelium

Alvear glioepithelium

Stem cells of the choroid plexus

Temporal neuroepithelium and subventricular zone

Caudate (tail)

Subpial granular layer

Posterior striatal neuroepithelium and subventricular zone

Temporal stratified transitional field

Lateral migratory stream
(infiltrating the claustrum and entering the insular cortex)

Germinal and transitional structures in *italics*

PLATE 47A
CR 235 mm
GW 26, Y16-59
Horizontal
Section 560

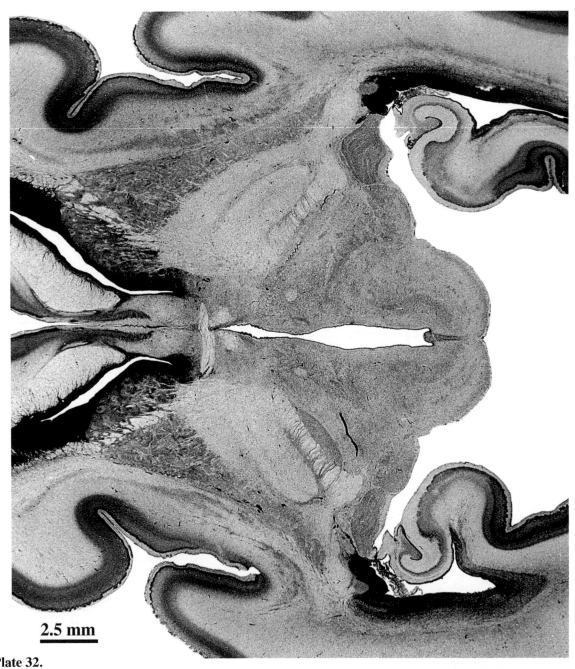

2.5 mm

See the entire Section 560 in Plate 32.

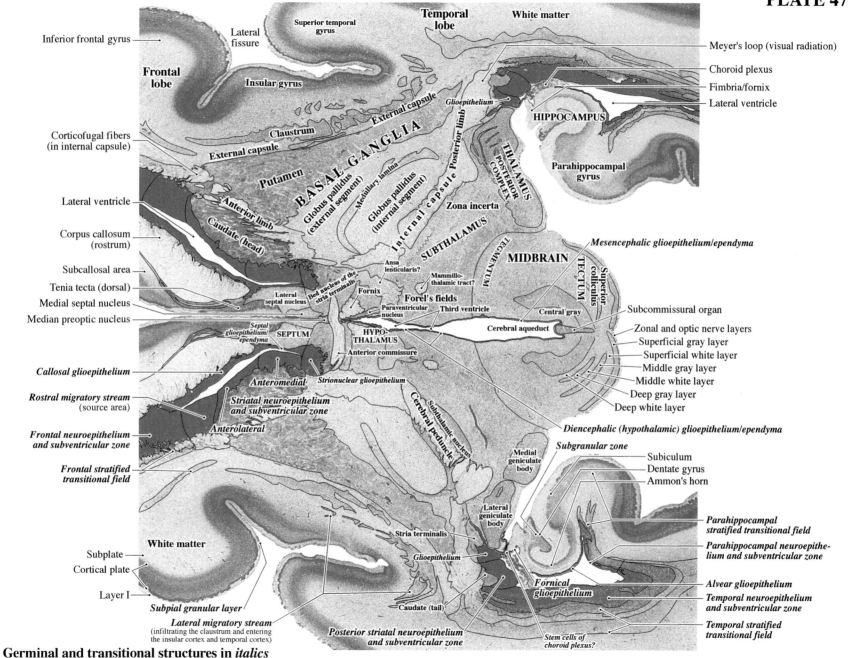

Inferior frontal gyrus

Lateral fissure

Superior temporal gyrus

Temporal lobe

White matter

Meyer's loop (visual radiation)

Choroid plexus

Fimbria/fornix

Lateral ventricle

Frontal lobe

Insular gyrus

Glioepithelium

HIPPOCAMPUS

Corticofugal fibers (in internal capsule)

External capsule

External capsule

Claustrum

External capsule

BASAL GANGLIA

Posterior limb

THALAMUS POSTERIOR COMPLEX

Parahippocampal gyrus

Putamen

Globus pallidus (external segment)

Medullary lamina

Globus pallidus (internal segment)

Internal capsule

Zona incerta

Anterior limb

Caudate (head)

SUBTHALAMUS

TEGMENTUM

MIDBRAIN

TECTUM

Superior colliculus

Lateral ventricle

Corpus callosum (rostrum)

Mesencephalic glioepithelium/ependyma

Ansa lenticularis?

Mammillo-thalamic tract?

Subcallosal area

Tenia tecta (dorsal)

Medial septal nucleus

Median preoptic nucleus

Bed nucleus of the stria terminalis

Lateral septal nucleus

Fornix

Forel's fields

Paraventricular nucleus

Third ventricle

Central gray

Subcommissural organ

Cerebral aqueduct

Zonal and optic nerve layers

Superficial gray layer

Superficial white layer

Middle gray layer

Middle white layer

Deep gray layer

Deep white layer

Septal glioepithelium/ ependyma

SEPTUM

HYPO-THALAMUS

Anterior commissure

Callosal glioepithelium

Anteromedial

Strionuclear glioepithelium

Rostral migratory stream (source area)

Striatal neuroepithelium and subventricular zone

Cerebral peduncle

Subthalamic nucleus

Diencephalic (hypothalamic) glioepithelium/ependyma

Frontal neuroepithelium and subventricular zone

Anterolateral

Subgranular zone

Medial geniculate body

Subiculum

Dentate gyrus

Ammon's horn

Frontal stratified transitional field

Lateral geniculate body

Parahippocampal stratified transitional field

White matter

Parahippocampal neuroepithelium and subventricular zone

Subplate

Cortical plate

Stria terminalis

Layer I

Glioepithelium

Alvear glioepithelium

Fornical glioepithelium

Temporal neuroepithelium and subventricular zone

Subpial granular layer

Caudate (tail)

Lateral migratory stream (infiltrating the claustrum and entering the insular cortex and temporal cortex)

Posterior striatal neuroepithelium and subventricular zone

Stem cells of choroid plexus?

Temporal stratified transitional field

Germinal and transitional structures in *italics*

100

PLATE 48A, CR 235 mm, GW 26, Y16-59
Horizontal, Section 620

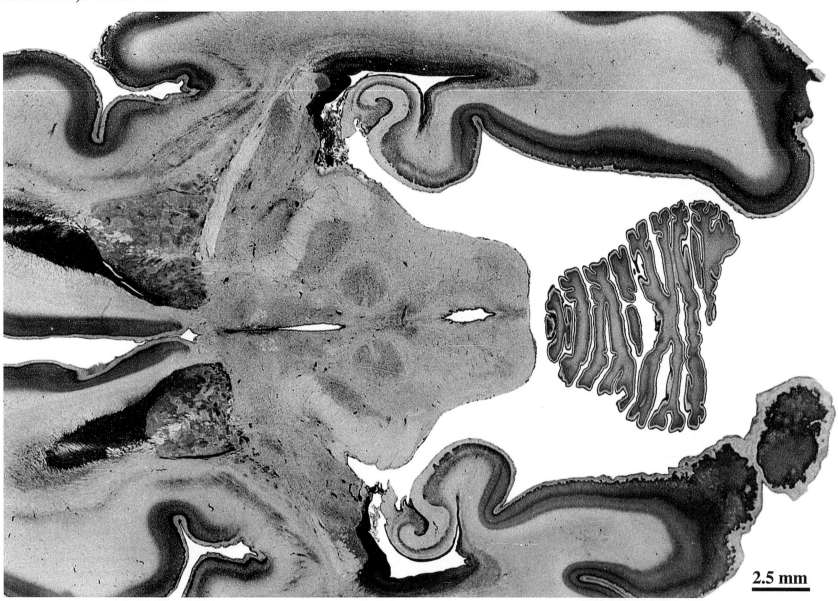

2.5 mm

See the entire Section 620 in Plate 33.

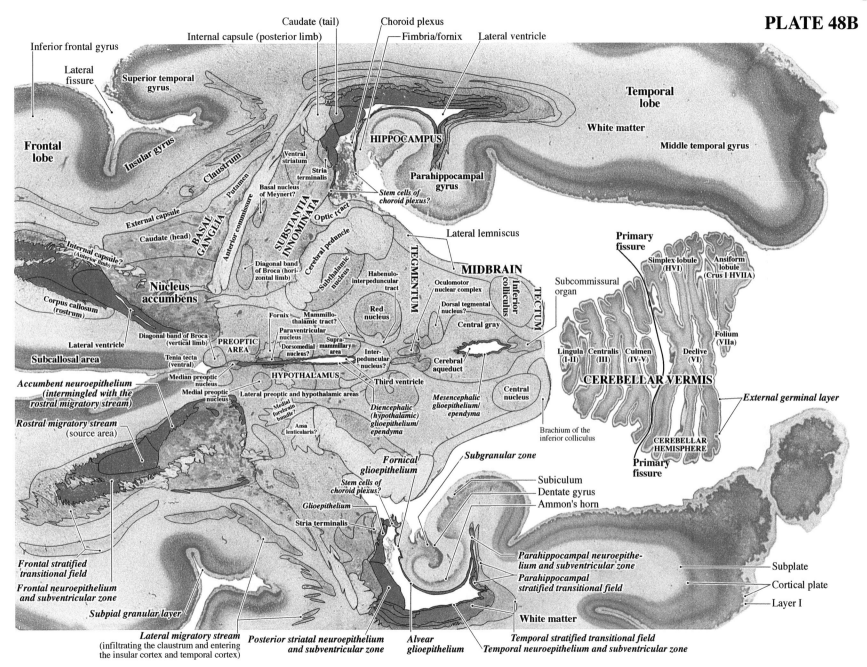

Inferior frontal gyrus

Lateral fissure

Superior temporal gyrus

Frontal lobe

Insular gyrus

Claustrum

External capsule

BASAL GANGLIA

Caudate (head)

Putamen

Anterior commissure

Internal capsule? *(Anterior limb)*

Corpus callosum (rostrum)

Nucleus accumbens

Lateral ventricle

Diagonal band of Broca (vertical limb)

Subcallosal area

Accumbent neuroepithelium (intermingled with the rostral migratory stream)

Rostral migratory stream (source area)

Frontal stratified transitional field

Frontal neuroepithelium and subventricular zone

Subpial granular layer

Lateral migratory stream (infiltrating the claustrum and entering the insular cortex and temporal cortex)

Caudate (tail)

Internal capsule (posterior limb)

Choroid plexus

Fimbria/fornix

Lateral ventricle

HIPPOCAMPUS

Ventral striatum

Stria terminalis

Basal nucleus of Meynert?

SUBSTANTIA INNOMINATA

Optic tract

Cerebral peduncle

Subthalamic nucleus

Diagonal band of Broca (horizontal limb)

PREOPTIC AREA

Fornix

Mammillothalamic tract?

Paraventricular nucleus

Dorsomedial nucleus?

Supramammillary area

Median preoptic nucleus

Medial preoptic nucleus

Tenia tecta (ventral)

HYPOTHALAMUS

Lateral preoptic and hypothalamic areas

Medial forebrain bundle?

Ansa lenticularis?

Stem cells of choroid plexus?

Temporal lobe

White matter

Middle temporal gyrus

Parahippocampal gyrus

Lateral lemniscus

TEGMENTUM

Habenulo-interpeduncular tract

MIDBRAIN

Oculomotor nuclear complex

Dorsal tegmental nucleus?

Central gray

Red nucleus

Interpeduncular nucleus?

Cerebral aqueduct

Third ventricle

Diencephalic (hypothalamic) glioepithelium/ ependyma

Mesencephalic glioepithelium/ ependyma

Subcommissural organ

Inferior colliculus

TECTUM

Central nucleus

Primary fissure

Simplex lobule (HVI)

Ansiform lobule (Crus I HVIIA)

Folium (VIIa)

Lingula (I-II)

Centralis (III)

Culmen (IV-V)

Declive (VI)

CEREBELLAR VERMIS

External germinal layer

Brachium of the inferior colliculus

Primary fissure

Subgranular zone

Fornical glioepithelium

Stem cells of choroid plexus?

Glioepithelium

Stria terminalis

CEREBELLAR HEMISPHERE

Subiculum

Dentate gyrus

Ammon's horn

Parahippocampal neuroepithelium and subventricular zone

Parahippocampal stratified transitional field

Subplate

Cortical plate

Layer I

White matter

Alvear glioepithelium

Posterior striatal neuroepithelium and subventricular zone

Temporal stratified transitional field

Temporal neuroepithelium and subventricular zone

Germinal and transitional structures in *italics*

PLATE 49A, CR 235 mm, GW 26, Y16-59
Horizontal, Section 660

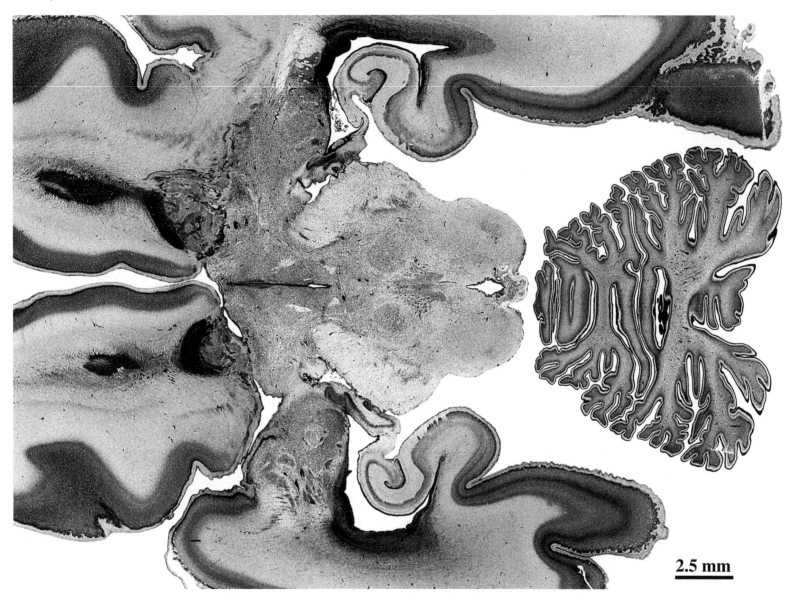

2.5 mm

See the entire Section 660 in Plate 34.

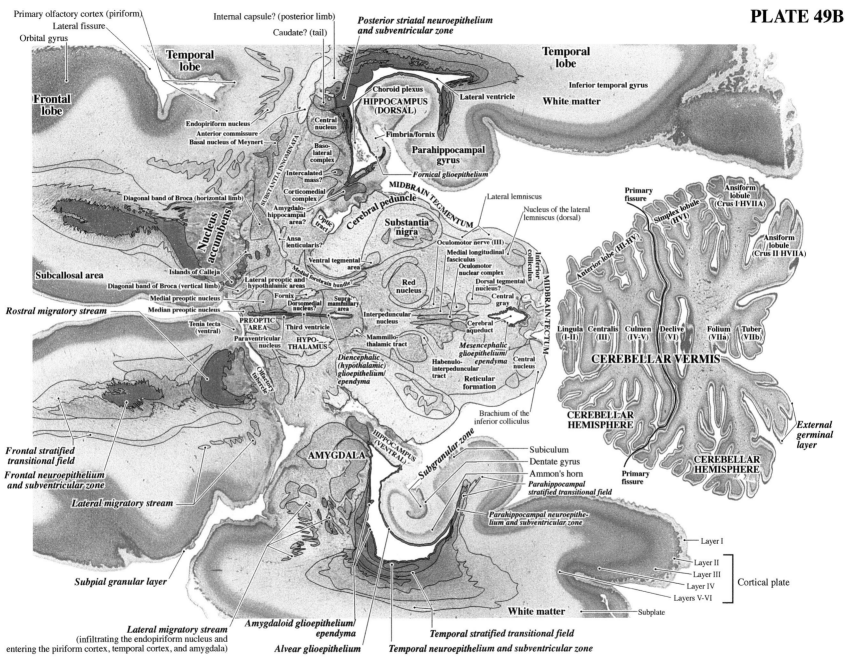

Primary olfactory cortex (piriform)
Lateral fissure
Orbital gyrus
Internal capsule? (posterior limb)
Caudate? (tail)
Posterior striatal neuroepithelium and subventricular zone
Temporal lobe
Choroid plexus
HIPPOCAMPUS (DORSAL)
Lateral ventricle
Temporal lobe
Inferior temporal gyrus
White matter
Frontal lobe
Endopiriform nucleus
Anterior commissure
Basal nucleus of Meynert
Central nucleus
Fimbria/fornix
Parahippocampal gyrus
Fornical glioepithelium
Baso-lateral complex
Intercalated mass?
Corticomedial complex
Amygdalo-hippocampal area?
SUBSTANTIA INNOMINATA
Diagonal band of Broca (horizontal limb)
MIDBRAIN TEGMENTUM
Cerebral peduncle
Lateral lemniscus
Nucleus of the lateral lemniscus (dorsal)
Optic tract
Substantia nigra
Nucleus accumbens
Ansa lenticularis?
Medial forebrain bundle?
Ventral tegmental area
Oculomotor nerve (III)
Medial longitudinal fasciculus
Oculomotor nuclear complex
Inferior colliculus
Subcallosal area
Islands of Calleja
Lateral preoptic and hypothalamic areas
Red nucleus
Dorsal tegmental nucleus?
Diagonal band of Broca (vertical limb)
Medial preoptic nucleus
Median preoptic nucleus
Fornix
Dorsomedial nucleus?
Supra-mammillary area
Central gray
MIDBRAIN TECTUM
Rostral migratory stream
Tenia tecta (ventral)
PREOPTIC AREA
Third ventricle
Interpeduncular nucleus
Cerebral aqueduct
Central nucleus
Paraventricular nucleus
HYPO-THALAMUS
Mammillo-thalamic tract
Mesencephalic glioepithelium ependyma
Diencephalic (hypothalamic) glioepithelium/ ependyma
Habenulo-interpeduncular tract
Central nucleus
Reticular formation
Lingula (I-II)
Centralis (III)
Culmen (IV-V)
Declive (VI)
Folium (VIIa)
Tuber (VIIb)
Olfactory tubercle
Brachium of the inferior colliculus
CEREBELLAR VERMIS
Frontal stratified transitional field
Frontal neuroepithelium and subventricular zone
CEREBELLAR HEMISPHERE
External germinal layer
HIPPOCAMPUS (VENTRAL)
Subiculum
Dentate gyrus
Subgranular zone
CEREBELLAR HEMISPHERE
Lateral migratory stream
AMYGDALA
Ammon's horn
Parahippocampal stratified transitional field
Primary fissure
Parahippocampal neuroepithelium and subventricular zone
Layer I
Layer II
Layer III
Layer IV
Layers V-VI
Cortical plate
Subpial granular layer
White matter
Subplate
Lateral migratory stream
(infiltrating the endopiriform nucleus and entering the piriform cortex, temporal cortex, and amygdala)
Amygdaloid glioepithelium/ ependyma
Temporal stratified transitional field
Alvear glioepithelium
Temporal neuroepithelium and subventricular zone
Primary fissure
Anterior lobe (HI-HV)
Simplex lobule (HVI)
Primary fissure
Ansiform lobule (Crus I HVIIA)
Ansiform lobule (Crus II HVIIA)

Germinal and transitional structures in *italics*

PLATE 50A, CR 235 mm, GW 26, Y16-59
Horizontal, Section 700

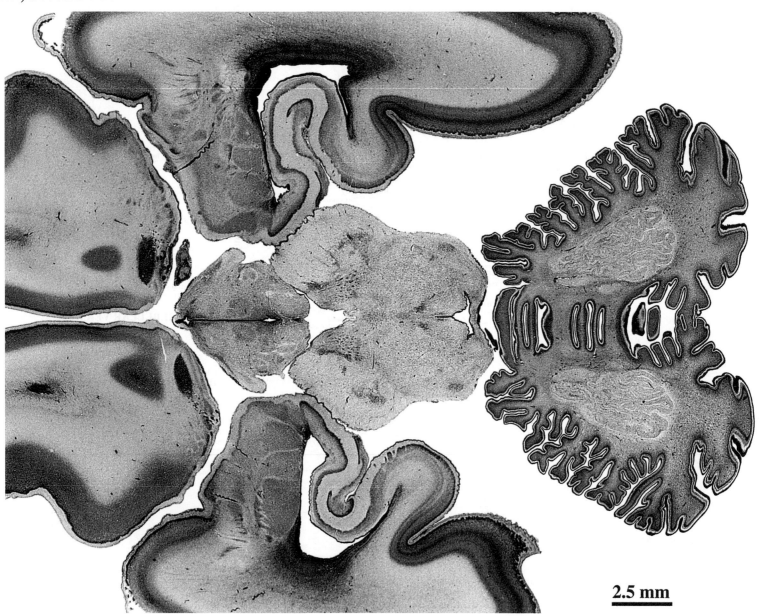

2.5 mm

See the entire Section 700 in Plate 35.

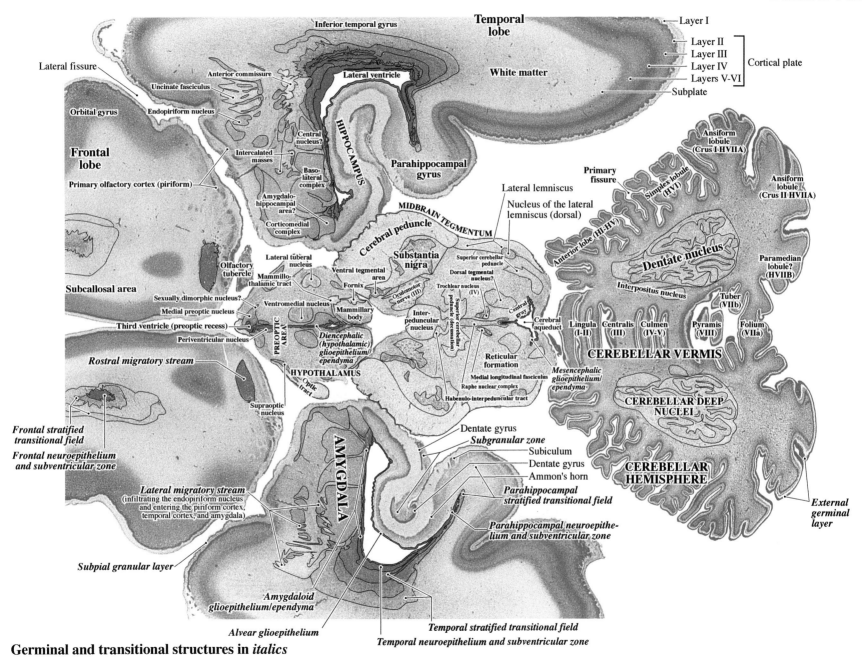

Germinal and transitional structures in *italics*

PLATE 51A, CR 235 mm, GW 26, Y16-59
Horizontal, Section 740

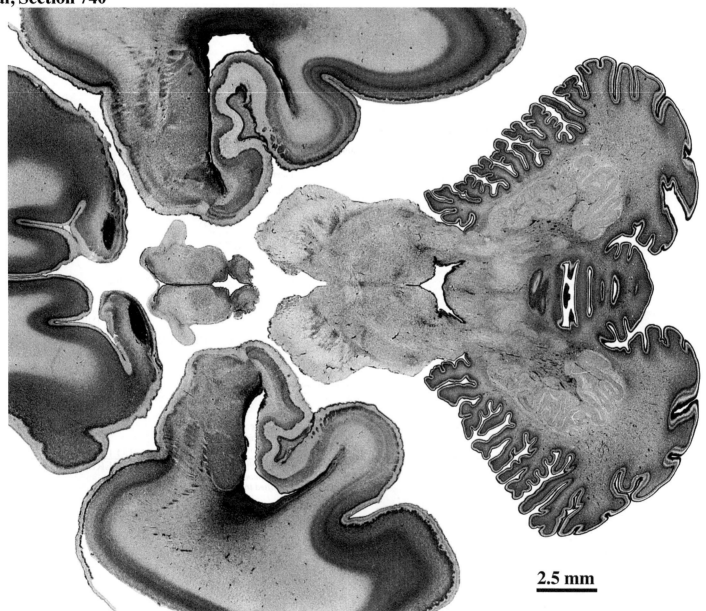

2.5 mm

See the entire Section 740 in Plate 36.

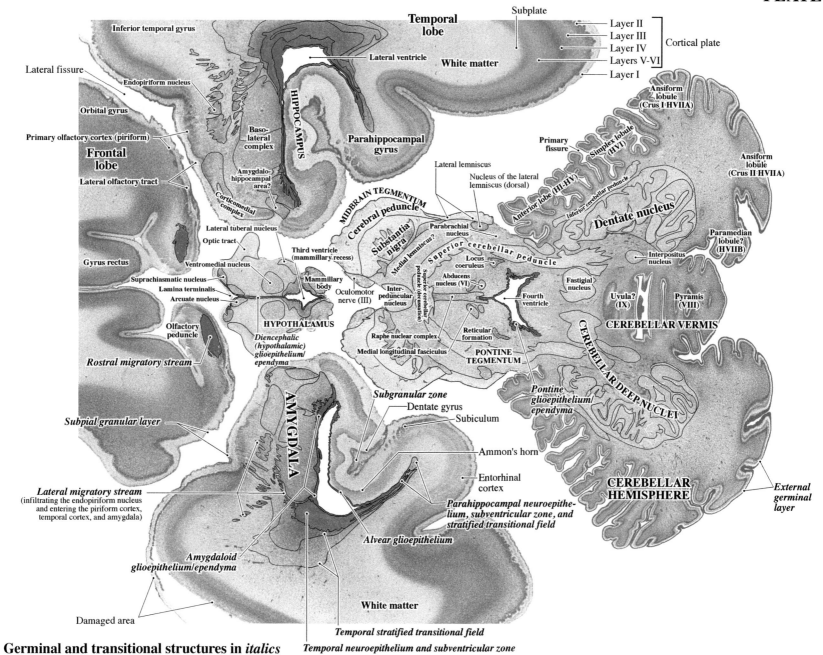

Inferior temporal gyrus

Temporal lobe

Subplate

Layer II
Layer III
Layer IV
Layers V-VI
Layer I

Cortical plate

Lateral ventricle

White matter

Lateral fissure

Endopiriform nucleus

Orbital gyrus

HIPPOCAMPUS

Ansiform lobule (Crus I HVIIA)

Primary olfactory cortex (piriform)

Baso-lateral complex

Parahippocampal gyrus

Primary fissure

Simplex lobule (HVI)

Ansiform lobule (Crus II HVIIA)

Frontal lobe

Amygdalo-hippocampal area?

Lateral lemniscus

Nucleus of the lateral lemniscus (dorsal)

Lateral olfactory tract

Corticomedial complex

MIDBRAIN TEGMENTUM

Cerebral peduncle

Parabrachial nucleus

Anterior lobe (HI-HV)

Inferior cerebellar peduncle

Dentate nucleus

Gyrus rectus

Lateral tuberal nucleus

Optic tract

Substantia nigra

Medial lemniscus?

Superior cerebellar peduncle

Paramedian lobule? (HVIIB)

Third ventricle (mammillary recess)

Superior cerebellar peduncle (decussation)

Locus coeruleus

Interpositus nucleus

Ventromedial nucleus

Suprachiasmatic nucleus

Mammillary body

Abducens nucleus (VI)

Fastigial nucleus

Lamina terminalis

Oculomotor nerve (III)

Inter-peduncular nucleus

Fourth ventricle

Uvula? (IX)

Pyramis (VIII)

Arcuate nucleus

Olfactory peduncle

HYPOTHALAMUS

Raphe nuclear complex

Reticular formation

CEREBELLAR VERMIS

Diencephalic (hypothalamic) glioepithelium/ ependyma

Medial longitudinal fasciculus

PONTINE TEGMENTUM

Rostral migratory stream

Subgranular zone

Pontine glioepithelium/ ependyma

CEREBELLAR DEEP NUCLEI

Dentate gyrus

Subpial granular layer

AMYGDALA

Subiculum

Ammon's horn

Entorhinal cortex

Lateral migratory stream
(infiltrating the endopiriform nucleus and entering the piriform cortex, temporal cortex, and amygdala)

Parahippocampal neuroepithelium, subventricular zone, and stratified transitional field

CEREBELLAR HEMISPHERE

External germinal layer

Alvear glioepithelium

Amygdaloid glioepithelium/ependyma

Damaged area

White matter

Temporal stratified transitional field

Temporal neuroepithelium and subventricular zone

Germinal and transitional structures in *italics*

PLATE 52A, CR 235 mm, GW 26, Y16-59
Horizontal, Section 780

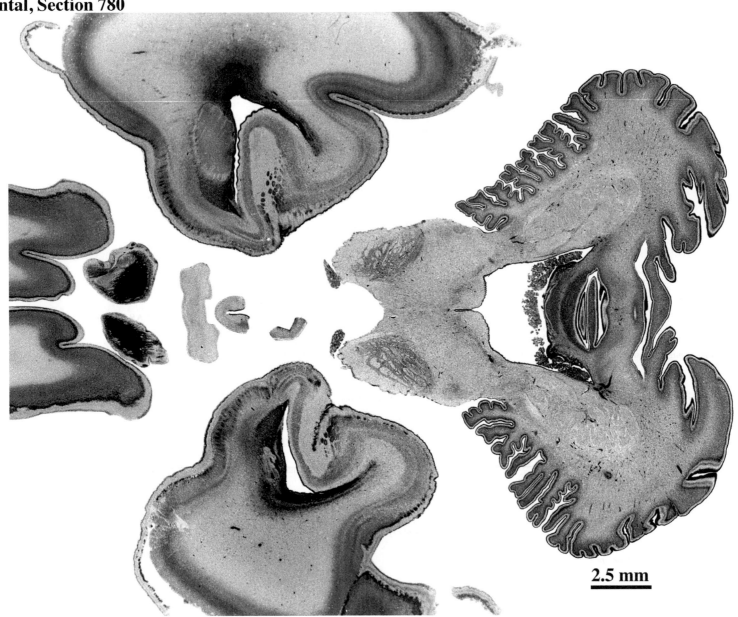

2.5 mm

See the entire Section 780 in Plate 37.

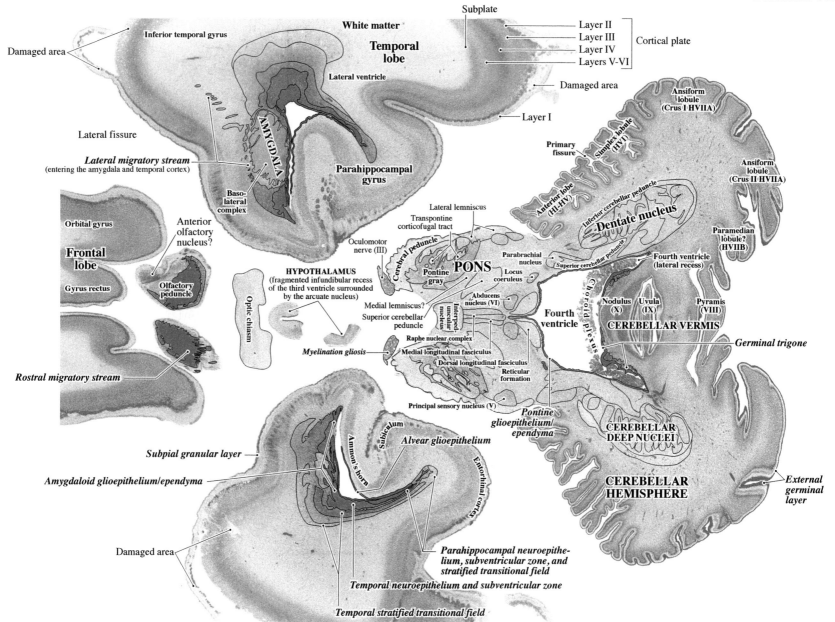

Inferior temporal gyrus

Damaged area

White matter

Temporal lobe

Subplate

Layer II
Layer III
Layer IV
Layers V-VI

Cortical plate

Lateral ventricle

Damaged area

Layer I

Ansiform lobule (Crus I HVIIA)

Lateral fissure

Simplex lobule (HVI)

Primary fissure

Ansiform lobule (Crus II HVIIA)

Lateral migratory stream
(entering the amygdala and temporal cortex)

AMYGDALA

Parahippocampal gyrus

Anterior lobe (HI-HV)

Inferior cerebellar peduncle

Dentate nucleus

Baso-lateral complex

Lateral lemniscus

Transpontine corticofugal tract

Paramedian lobule? (HVIIB)

Orbital gyrus

Anterior olfactory nucleus?

Oculomotor nerve (III)

Cerebral peduncle

Parabrachial nucleus

Superior cerebellar peduncle

Fourth ventricle (lateral recess)

Frontal lobe

Pontine gray

PONS

Locus coeruleus

Gyrus rectus

Olfactory peduncle

HYPOTHALAMUS
(fragmented infundibular recess of the third ventricle surrounded by the arcuate nucleus)

Medial lemniscus?

Superior cerebellar peduncle

Abducens nucleus (VI)

Interpeduncular nucleus

Fourth ventricle

Choroid plexus

Nodulus (X)

Uvula (IX)

Pyramis (VIII)

Optic chiasm

Myelination gliosis

Rostral migratory stream

Raphe nuclear complex
Medial longitudinal fasciculus
Dorsal longitudinal fasciculus
Reticular formation

CEREBELLAR VERMIS

Germinal trigone

Principal sensory nucleus (V)

Pontine glioepithelium/ependyma

Subpial granular layer

Subiculum

Alvear glioepithelium

Ammon's horn

Amygdaloid glioepithelium/ependyma

Entorhinal cortex

CEREBELLAR DEEP NUCLEI

CEREBELLAR HEMISPHERE

External germinal layer

Damaged area

Parahippocampal neuroepithelium, subventricular zone, and stratified transitional field

Temporal neuroepithelium and subventricular zone

Temporal stratified transitional field

Germinal and transitional structures in *italics*

110

PLATE 53A, CR 235 mm, GW 26, Y16-59
Horizontal, Section 820

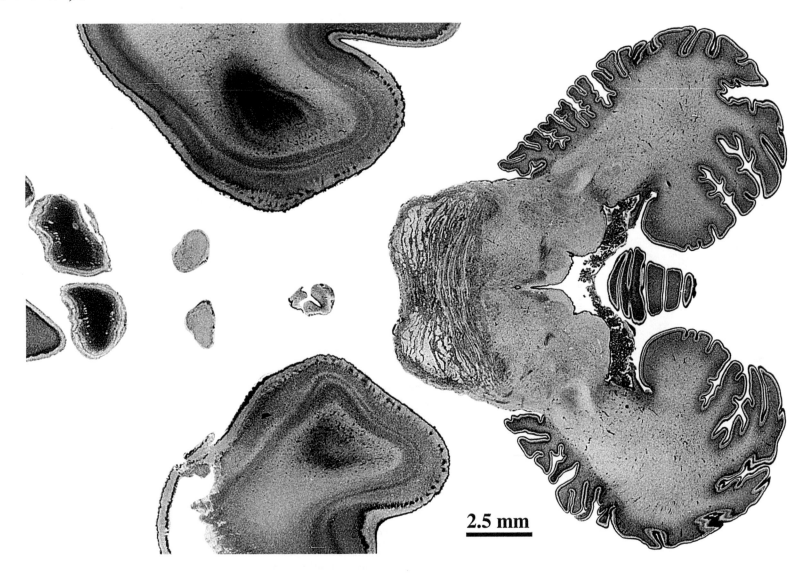

2.5 mm

See the entire Section 820 in Plate 38.

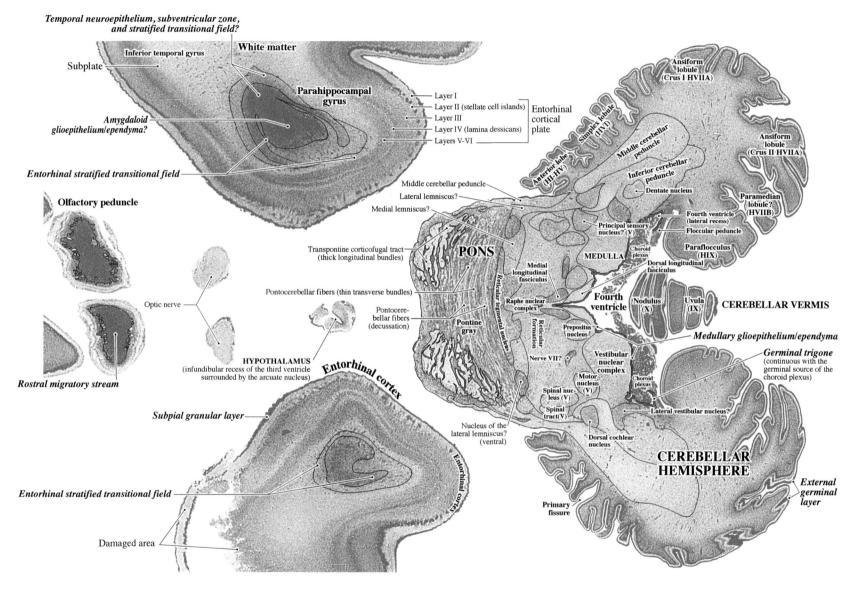

Temporal neuroepithelium, subventricular zone,
and stratified transitional field?

Inferior temporal gyrus

White matter

Subplate

**Parahippocampal
gyrus**

*Amygdaloid
glioepithelium/ependyma?*

Layer I
Layer II (stellate cell islands)
Layer III
Layer IV (lamina dessicans)
Layers V-VI

Entorhinal
cortical
plate

Entorhinal stratified transitional field

Olfactory peduncle

Optic nerve

Rostral migratory stream

Middle cerebellar peduncle

Lateral lemniscus?

Medial lemniscus?

Transpontine corticofugal tract
(thick longitudinal bundles)

Pontocerebellar fibers (thin transverse bundles)

Pontocere-
bellar fibers
(decussation)

PONS

**Pontine
gray**

Medial
longitudinal
fasciculus

Reticular tegmental nucleus

Raphe nuclear
complex

Reticular
formation

Nerve VII?

Nucleus of the
lateral lemniscus?
(ventral)

HYPOTHALAMUS
(infundibular recess of the third ventricle
surrounded by the arcuate nucleus)

Entorhinal cortex

Subpial granular layer

Entorhinal stratified transitional field

Damaged area

Entorhinal cortex

**Ansiform
lobule
(Crus I HVIIA)**

Simplex lobule
(HVI)

Middle cerebellar
peduncle

**Ansiform
lobule
(Crus II HVIIA)**

Anterior lobe
(HI-HV)

Inferior cerebellar
peduncle

Dentate nucleus

**Paramedian
lobule?
(HVIIB)**

Principal sensory
nucleus? (V)

Fourth ventricle
(lateral recess)

Floccular peduncle

MEDULLA

Choroid
plexus

Dorsal longitudinal
fasciculus

**Paraflocculus
(HIX)**

**Fourth
ventricle**

Prepositus
nucleus

Nodulus
(X)

Uvula
(IX)

CEREBELLAR VERMIS

Medullary glioepithelium/ependyma

Germinal trigone
(continuous with the
germinal source of the
choroid plexus)

Vestibular
nuclear
complex

Motor
nucleus
(V)

Choroid
plexus

Spinal nuc-
leus (V)

Spinal
tract (V)

Lateral vestibular nucleus?

Dorsal cochlear
nucleus

**CEREBELLAR
HEMISPHERE**

*External
germinal
layer*

Primary
fissure

Germinal and transitional structures in *italics*

112

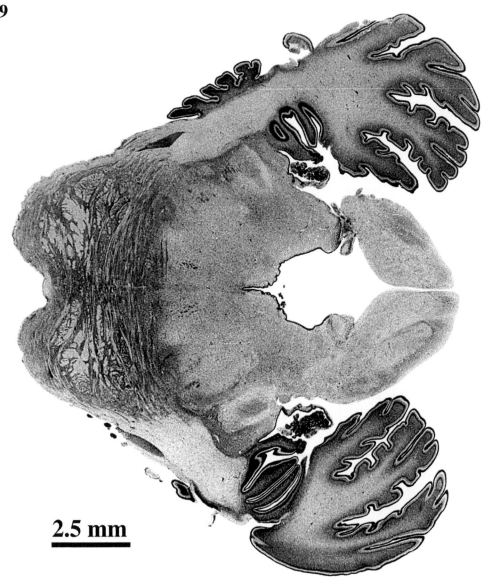

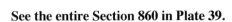

2.5 mm

See the entire Section 860 in Plate 39.

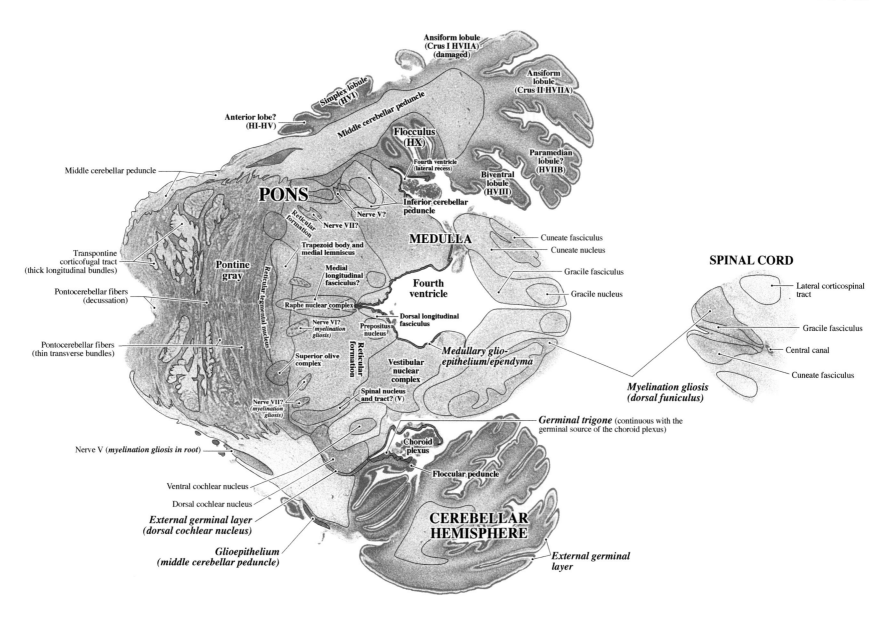

Ansiform lobule
(Crus I HVIIA)
(damaged)

Ansiform
lobule
(Crus II·HVIIA)

Simplex lobule
(HVI)

Anterior lobe?
(HI–HV)

Middle cerebellar peduncle

Flocculus
(HX)

Paramedian
lobule?
(HVIIB)

Middle cerebellar peduncle

Fourth ventricle
(lateral recess)

Biventral
lobule
(HVIII)

PONS

Reticular
formation

Nerve V?

Inferior cerebellar
peduncle

Nerve VII?

MEDULLA

Cuneate fasciculus

Cuneate nucleus

Trapezoid body and
medial lemniscus

Reticular tegmental nucleus

Transpontine
corticofugal tract
(thick longitudinal bundles)

**Pontine
gray**

Medial
longitudinal
fasciculus?

Gracile fasciculus

Pontocerebellar fibers
(decussation)

**Fourth
ventricle**

Gracile nucleus

SPINAL CORD

Raphe nuclear complex

Lateral corticospinal
tract

Nerve VI?
*(myelination
gliosis)*

Dorsal longitudinal
fasciculus

Prepositus
nucleus

Reticular
formation

Pontocerebellar fibers
(thin transverse bundles)

Gracile fasciculus

*Medullary glio-
epithelium/ependyma*

Superior olive
complex

Vestibular
nuclear
complex

Central canal

Cuneate fasciculus

Nerve VII?
*(myelination
gliosis)*

Spinal nucleus
and tract? (V)

*Myelination gliosis
(dorsal funiculus)*

Nerve V *(myelination gliosis in root)*

Germinal trigone (continuous with the
germinal source of the choroid plexus)

*Choroid
plexus*

Ventral cochlear nucleus

Dorsal cochlear nucleus

Floccular
peduncle

*External germinal layer
(dorsal cochlear nucleus)*

**CEREBELLAR
HEMISPHERE**

*Glioepithelium
(middle cerebellar peduncle)*

*External germinal
layer*

Germinal and transitional structures in *italics*

114

PLATE 55A
CR 235 mm
GW 26, Y16-59
Horizontal
Section 880

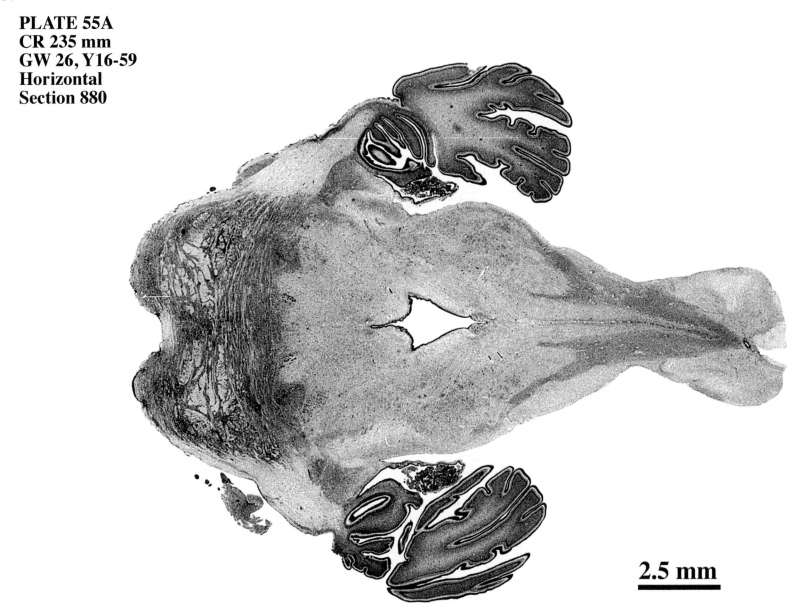

2.5 mm

See the entire Section 880 in Plate 40.

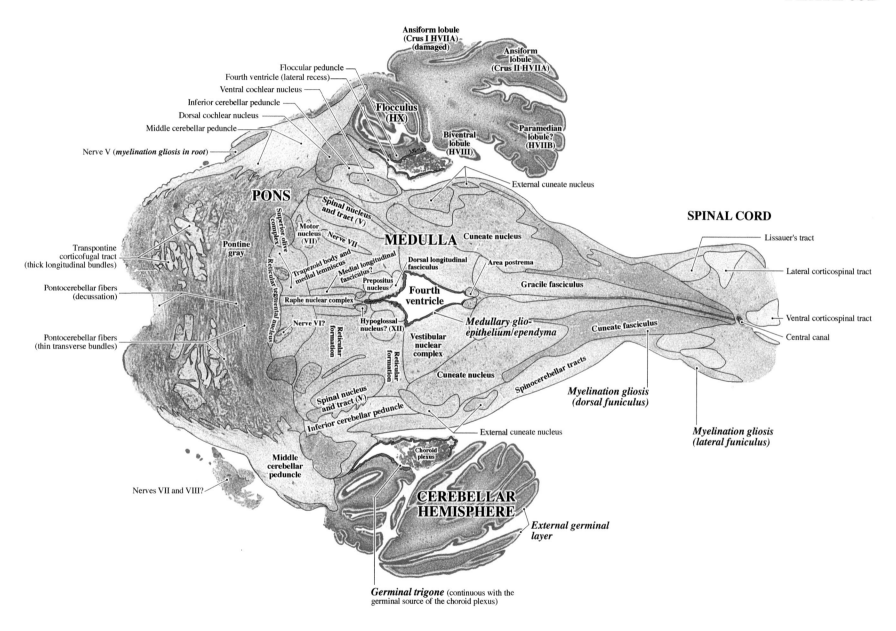

Ansiform lobule
(Crus I HVIIA)
(damaged)

Ansiform lobule
(Crus II HVIIA)

Floccular peduncle
Fourth ventricle (lateral recess)
Ventral cochlear nucleus
Inferior cerebellar peduncle
Dorsal cochlear nucleus
Middle cerebellar peduncle

**Flocculus
(HX)**

**Biventral
lobule
(HVIII)**

Paramedian
lobule?
(HVIIB)

Nerve V (*myelination gliosis in root*)

External cuneate nucleus

PONS

*Spinal nucleus
and tract (V)*

SPINAL CORD

Superior olive
complex

Motor
nucleus
(VII)

Nerve VII

MEDULLA

Cuneate nucleus

Lissauer's tract

Transpontine
corticofugal tract
(thick longitudinal bundles)

**Pontine
gray**

Reticular tegmental nucleus

Trapezoid body and
medial lemniscus

Medial longitudinal
fasciculus

Prepositus
nucleus?

Dorsal longitudinal
fasciculus

Area postrema

Lateral corticospinal tract

Gracile fasciculus

Pontocerebellar fibers
(decussation)

Raphe nuclear complex

Prepositus
nucleus

**Fourth
ventricle**

*Medullary glio-
epithelium/ependyma*

Cuneate fasciculus

Ventral corticospinal tract

Pontocerebellar fibers
(thin transverse bundles)

Nerve VI?

Reticular
formation

Hypoglossal
nucleus? (XII)

Reticular
formation

**Vestibular
nuclear
complex**

Central canal

Spinocerebellar tracts

*Myelination gliosis
(dorsal funiculus)*

Cuneate nucleus

*Spinal nucleus
and tract (V)*

Inferior cerebellar peduncle

External cuneate nucleus

*Myelination gliosis
(lateral funiculus)*

Choroid
plexus

**Middle
cerebellar
peduncle**

Nerves VII and VIII?

**CEREBELLAR
HEMISPHERE**

*External germinal
layer*

Germinal trigone (continuous with the
germinal source of the choroid plexus)

Germinal and transitional structures in *italics*

PLATE 56A
CR 235 mm
GW 26, Y16-59
Horizontal
Section 900

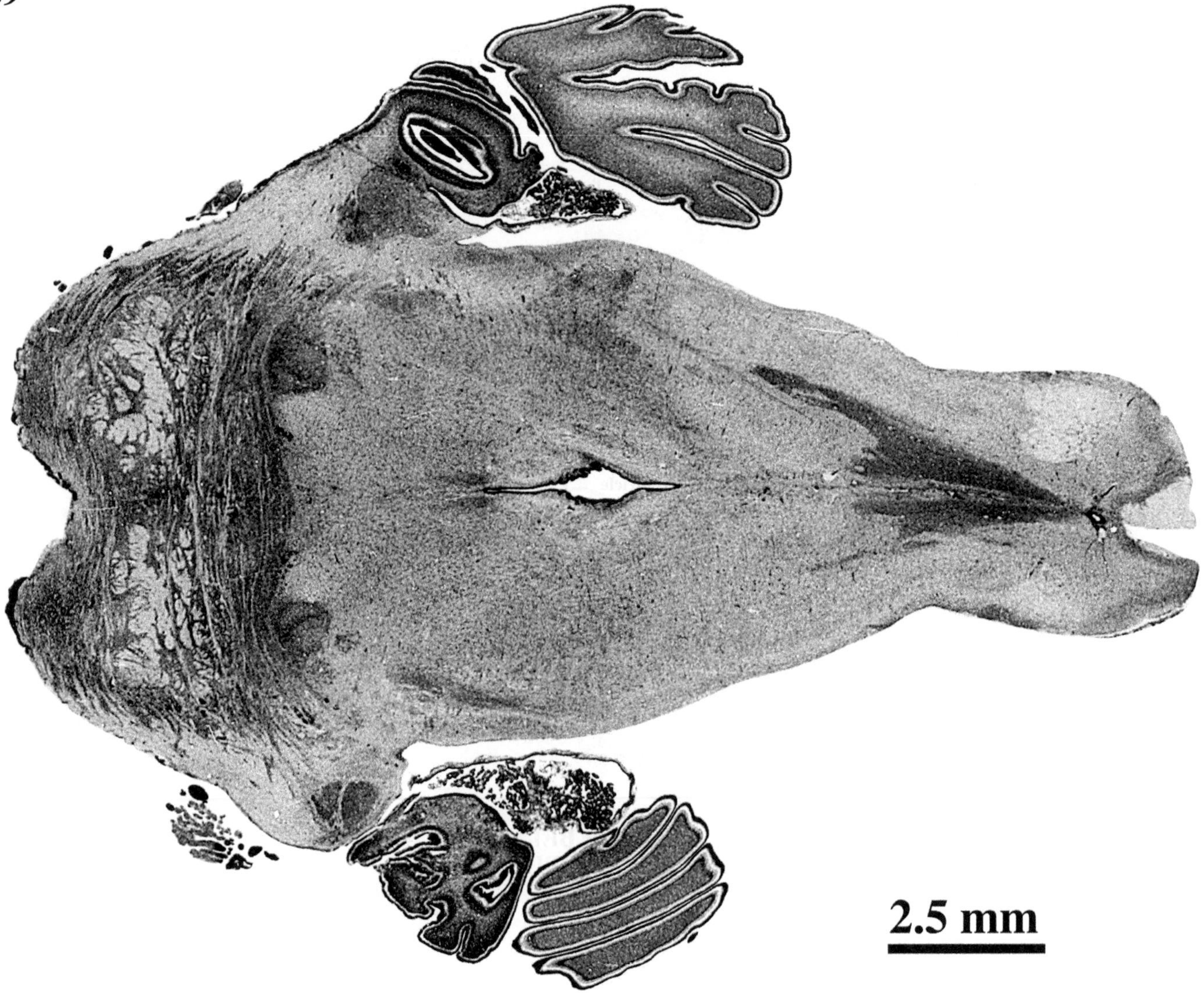

2.5 mm

See the entire Section 900 in Plate 41.

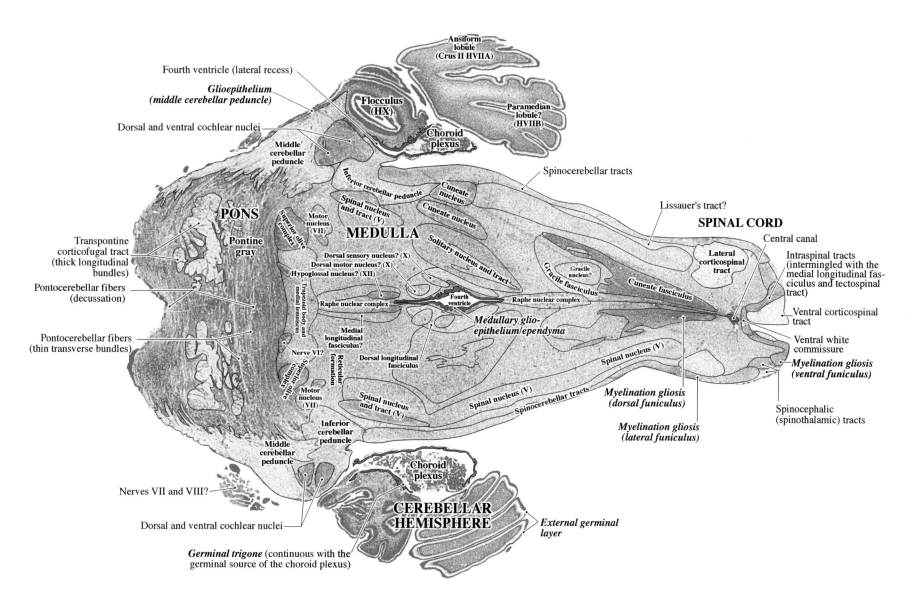

Ansiform
lobule
(Crus II HVIIA)

Fourth ventricle (lateral recess)

***Glioepithelium
(middle cerebellar peduncle)***

Flocculus
(HX)

Paramedian
lobule?
(HVIIB)

Dorsal and ventral cochlear nuclei

Choroid
plexus

Middle
cerebellar
peduncle

Spinocerebellar tracts

Inferior cerebellar peduncle

Cuneate
nucleus

Cuneate nucleus

Spinal nucleus
and tract (V)

PONS

Motor
nucleus
(VII)

Lissauer's tract?

SPINAL CORD

Superior olive complex

Pontine
gray

MEDULLA

Solitary nucleus and tract

Central canal

Transpontine
corticofugal tract
(thick longitudinal
bundles)

Dorsal sensory nucleus? (X)
Dorsal motor nucleus? (X)
Hypoglossal nucleus? (XII)

Lateral
corticospinal
tract

Intraspinal tracts
(intermingled with the
medial longitudinal fas-
ciculus and tectospinal
tract)

Gracile
nucleus?

Gracile fasciculus

Cuneate fasciculus

Pontocerebellar fibers
(decussation)

Raphe nuclear complex

Fourth
ventricle

Raphe nuclear complex

Ventral corticospinal
tract

Trapezoid body and medial lemniscus

Medial
longitudinal
fasciculus?

***Medullary glio-
epithelium/ependyma***

Ventral white
commissure

Pontocerebellar fibers
(thin transverse bundles)

Nerve VI?

Reticular formation

Dorsal longitudinal
fasciculus

Spinal nucleus (V)

***Myelination gliosis
(ventral funiculus)***

Superior olive complex

Motor
nucleus
(VII)

Spinal nucleus
and tract (V)

Spinal nucleus (V)

***Myelination gliosis
(dorsal funiculus)***

Spinocephalic
(spinothalamic) tracts

Inferior
cerebellar
peduncle

Spinocerebellar tracts

***Myelination gliosis
(lateral funiculus)***

Middle
cerebellar
peduncle

Choroid
plexus

Nerves VII and VIII?

**CEREBELLAR
HEMISPHERE**

***External germinal
layer***

Dorsal and ventral cochlear nuclei

Germinal trigone (continuous with the
germinal source of the choroid plexus)

Germinal and transitional structures in *italics*